The Menopause Revolution: Smashing the HRT Myth

Natural Alternatives to Manufactured Drug Therapy

Martin Milner N.D.

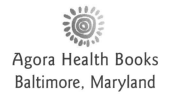

Agora Health Books
Baltimore, Maryland

680B001425

Martin Milner N.D.:
The Menopause Revolution: Smashing the HRT Myth

Published by Agora Health Books

Alice Wessendorf, Managing editor
Ken Danz, Copy editor

Copyright 2005 by Agora Health Books
All Rights Reserved

ISBN 1-891434-20-9

Printed in the United States of America
Cover and book design by Gerrit Wessendorf

Agora Health Books
819 N. Charles Street
Baltimore, Maryland 21201
www.agorahealthbooks.com

For additional copies of this book call 1-888-821-3609.

No part of this book, unless otherwise noted, may be copied or reproduced by any means or for any reason without the written consent of the publisher. The information contained herein is obtained from sources believed to be reliable, but its accuracy cannot be guaranteed.

Permission is granted to copy, distribute and/or modify illustrations provided by Wikipedia (www.wikipedia.org) in this document under the terms of the GNU Free Documentation License, Version 1.2 or any later version published by the Free Software Foundation; with no Invariant Sections, no Front-Cover Texts, and no Back-Cover Texts.

The Menopause Revolution: Smashing the HRT Myth
Natural Alternatives to Manufactured Drug Therapy

Martin Milner N.D.

Agora Health Books
Baltimore, Maryland

DISCLAIMER

All material in this publication is provided for information only and may not be construed as medical advice or instruction. No action should be taken based solely on the contents of this publication; instead, readers should consult appropriate health professionals on any matter relating to their health and well-being.

The information and opinions provided in this book are believed to be accurate and sound, based on the best judgment available to the authors, but readers who fail to consult with appropriate health authorities assume the risk of any injuries. The publisher is not responsible for errors or omissions.

THE INFORMATION PRESENTED HERE HAS NOT BEEN EVALUATED BY THE U.S. FOOD & DRUG ADMINISTRATION. THIS PRODUCT IS NOT INTENDED TO DIAGNOSE, TREAT, CURE, OR PREVENT ANY DISEASE.

Table of Contents

Dedication

This book is dedicated to my sister, Alice Cutler, who lives her life in service to so many people in so many ways. Ali went through menopause during a period of great personal and professional trial in her life. In spite of many challenges she was able to rise into deeper levels of personal power and self-awareness. She gained phenomenal insight into much of what life is all about—love, service, family, true friendship, and personal fulfillment. When it was all over, she looked back and realized menopause was behind her and she had moved through it naturally without drugs and with poise, grace, and personal integrity. She is a model to men and women everywhere. May we all move through life's challenges and pauses with heightened self-awareness.

Preface

Dear Reader,

Beware! You are holding a dangerous book in your hands. It's dangerous because it challenges much of the conventional wisdom behind the most common medical solutions offered to women going through menopause.

I have practiced medicine for 22 years and have prescribed drugs as well as natural medicine to address the symptoms of menopause. During this period, I have come across hundreds of women who, simply put, have been done a disservice by conventional medicine. They've either been prescribed powerful drugs that they don't need or been dosed in an imbalanced fashion without proper monitoring of levels by practitioners who haven't taken the time to devise a more conscientious course of treatment. In my opinion, this is criminal.

Too many women are falling prey to the "small-box" thinking that currently plagues the medical industry. During a checkup or an office visit for some other matter, they (maybe even you) might mention they're experiencing some menopausal symptoms. Without so much as a second thought, their doctors whip out their pads and prescribe standard doses of estrogen (often not biologically identical to human estrogens)—with or without synthetic progesterone. A few months later, everything's fine. The symptoms have gone away and the hormones are obviously working. That's good news, right? WRONG! Without checking to see what effect these hormones are actually having, how they are being metabolized, and what levels have accumulated, it's folly to arrive at this conclusion. Yet, most medical practitioners do just this, prescribe 0.625 mg of Premarin (conjugated estrogen), and if your symptoms clear up, they reason, you are fine.

It is ludicrous to prescribe powerful hormones without monitoring blood or 24-hour urine levels, but this is exactly what happens with too many women.

Another travesty takes place when hormones like Premarin are given to a woman who has lost her uterus and ovaries through hysterectomy. Her physician tells her that Premarin is safe; that it can't cause endometrial cancer because she doesn't have a uterus anymore. She takes Premarin for years and isn't monitored for levels of all estrogens and their metabolites. Unfortunately, she develops breast cancer. The tumor is biopsied, and the estrogen-receptor status analyzed. The results usually come back estrogen receptor positive. This same physician, out of the other side of his mouth, will be telling this patient to stop taking Premarin immediately.

I believe that most practitioners of conventional medicine are talented and intelligent people who, for a variety of reasons, have abdicated their common sense and become boxed into a narrowly defined regimen of practice that is more driven by economics, an antiquated hierarchy of knowledge cloaked in the hospital mega-complex, and special interests than anything else. As a consumer of medical services, this probably comes as no surprise to you; it has been going on for so long, however, that you may not remember what it is like to have a real therapeutic relationship with a physician.

These days, most patients are lucky if they spend more than a few minutes in a room with the "family doctor." They're luckier still if they spend those few minutes with the same person they saw the last time they went to the doctor's office. The sacred trust between patient and physician that used to be the heart and soul of the medical profession has been eroded to the point where it hardly exists anymore.

The once essential triangle formed by the patient, the physician, and the pharmacist has been eroded as well. This triangle serves as a check and balance system to ensure proper prescribing on the physician's part and proper educating and dispensing of medications on the pharmacist's part. These days, managed care has often circumvented this triangle with mail-order pharmacies and with patients taking multiple prescription drugs while having no personal relationship with a pharmacist. The basics of what makes a solid patient–physician–pharmacist relationship is often lost in the name of escalating health-care costs. In reality, this breakdown is costing the public many more health care dollars in drug-interaction side effects and drug-related health complications than it is saving.

More and more, consumers are taking matters into their own hands—literally—by buying books like this one and determining their own courses of action when it comes to their medical care. They're being forced into doing so, either by the high costs of conventional medical care or the discouragingly low levels of care they receive otherwise. It's no wonder that more and more people are sidestepping both physicians and pharmacists—who, by tradition, have also been part of that sacred trust—and are getting their prescriptions by mail. After all, a nameless, faceless "virtual" physician isn't much worse than the care that they're subjected to in a brick-and-mortar doctor's office.

As you can see, I am passionate about medicine—or, perhaps I should say, conscientious medicine. I am committed to the kind of medical practice that treats the whole body, that honors the relationships between the world in which we live and the things that sustain and nourish us, physically, mentally, and spiritually. A medical practice that is guided by the inherent wisdom found in nature. A medicine that uses natural substances and biologically identical hormones to replace deficiency states. I believe that the consumers of medical services deserve nothing less. YOU deserve nothing less.

Medicine began with inquiry, in asking why certain substances—plants and herbs—could affect healing when others did not. There is still much to be learned from the realm of natural medicine, in working with what the universe has provided us, yet conventional medicine has tossed aside much of it in the name of "science." This, too, is wrong. While science has its place, we must exercise great caution when we alter the molecular structure of hormones and dispense them in large quantities and significant doses to women across an entire culture. Recent research has shown that unnatural, molecularly altered estrogens and progesterones not found in the human body are not safe, in spite of 30 years of prior so-called medical science. Do we need more research to prove the obvious? If we stray from natural law and biologically identical hormones these medications will do damage sooner or later. The body isn't built to sustain a continuous chemical onslaught from multiple synthetic drugs and, of course, it shouldn't need to, if there is a known, safer, bio-identical alternative. The United States Food and Drug Association (FDA) licenses drugs after it determines them to be "safe" and effective. However, adverse health outcomes from drugs can take years to develop. This, as you will see below, is apparently the case with estrogen derived from the urine of pregnant horses (Premarin) and synthetic progesterone (medroxyprogesterone acetate).

This book is dangerous because it dares to present some alternatives to treating menopause that practitioners of conventional medicine rarely even consider. I believe it's necessary to put the broad array of treatments into perspective by giving you a rational, balanced discussion of all approaches—conventional and complementary—and you'll find this in the pages that follow as well. However, you will also see a great deal here about treatments you may not know much, if anything, about—specifically, the use of natural hormones that are a better physical match with a woman's own innate hormone production, and how those hormones can be customized to match each woman's specific needs through just a couple of simple tests.

Putting all of this information in your hands is important, because the approach you take to manage your menopause is ultimately up to you. Every woman's experiences, desires, and needs for this time in her life are different, and no one course of treatment will work for all. Because of this, no one else can—or should—make your decisions for you.

You've probably been told more than once that you have to be your own best advocate in order to receive the best medical care. To find the best treatment for your specific needs as you travel through menopause, however, you'll have to be more than an advocate. Getting to where you need to be will take some thinking outside of the box on your part as well. It may not be easy—in fact, it probably won't be—but if you're up to the challenge, you'll find that this particular journey is worth it. But, and here's the good news, those alternatives are easier to access than you may think.

Much of the impetus behind this book came from the findings of the Women's Health Initiative studies that were released in summer 2002. Those findings—that estrogen and progestin taken together for more than a few years will actually increase a woman's risk of developing potentially deadly cardiovascular problems, breast cancer, and osteoporosis, among other things—were so striking that the study was halted three years before its scheduled completion. For the first time, the medical community, as well as millions of women, had concrete answers regarding the endless debate over the efficacy of long-term conjugated estrogen (Premarin) from horse mare's urine and synthetic-progesterone hormone replacement therapy, and they clearly weren't good.

Those results angered and confused many women who had been led to believe that hormone replacement therapy is the gold standard when it comes to managing the symptoms of menopause and guarding against future health problems. It also left them with the sense that there are no viable alternatives to such therapy. There are, of course, many viable alternatives, and I have been offering them to my patients for years. It is imperative that we increase both the awareness of these alternatives and our access to them.

My hope is that you'll use this book to become, for lack of a better term, a menopause warrior. For, in some respects, getting the right care will be somewhat of a battle. I intend to walk you through the process every step of the way—to serve as your war council, so to speak—as we have a shared goal: your good health, both now and in the years to come. Together, we can accomplish it.

I wish you good health,

Dr. Martin Milner
Naturopathic Physician

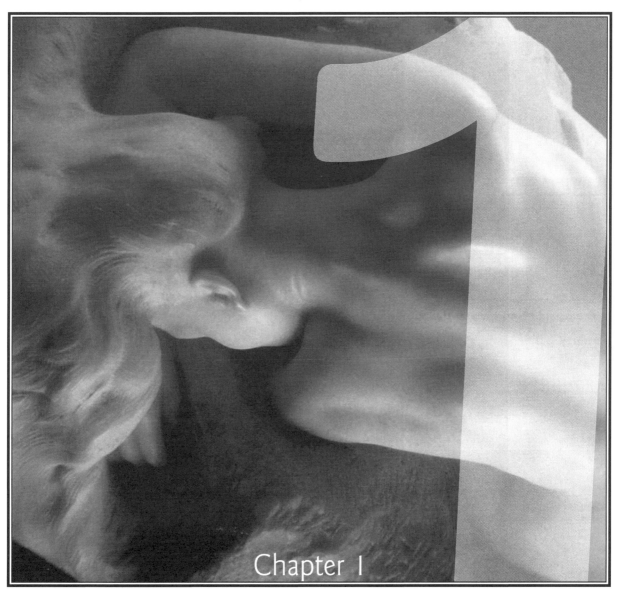

Chapter 1

Understanding Menopause

Chapter 1
Understanding Menopause

There are few sure things in a woman's life, but menopause* is one of them. This rite of passage, which marks the end of the childbearing years, is the shared link uniting all women, regardless of race, heritage, genes, or any other factors.

For being such a natural and inevitable part of a woman's life, menopause still carries a fairly strong stigma about it. In her landmark best seller <u>The Silent Passage</u>, published in 1992, author Gail Sheehy described menopause as "the last taboo" and decried both the overwhelming lack of information about it and the fact that most women were, in her words, "menophobic"—they had little desire to know more about this important stage of their lives, wanted even less to talk about it, and sometimes even shunned other women who were exhibiting obvious signs of going through the "change of life."

While more attention has been focused on menopause in recent years, it still continues to

* The term "menopause" is somewhat of a misnomer, as it technically describes just one day in a woman's life: the day that marks her having gone for 12 months without a period. Everything leading up to that day is technically perimenopause. Everything after that day is postmenopause. So when we talk about "going through menopause," we are actually talking about these two stages rather than the actual act of reaching menopause itself. Still, with the difference between the two phases being as short as a blink of an eye, they are generally lumped together under the umbrella term. Since this is what most people are familiar with, it's what I'll use in all general discussions in this book. The terms "perimenopause" and "postmenopause" will be used in discussions specifically dealing with these stages.

be an off-limits subject to varying degrees. These days, it seems as though few people have much problem going into minute details about almost every facet of their lives; yet menopause is still a touchy topic. Because of this, many women remain ill-informed about it or suffer with its problems in silence.

Menopause Terms

Menopause: the end of menstruation, confirmed after 12 consecutive months without a period or when the ovaries are removed or damaged

Perimenopause: the transitional time of up to six years or more immediately prior to natural menopause when changes begin, plus one year after menopause

Induced menopause: the immediate menopause caused by a medical or surgical intervention that removes or damages the ovaries

Premature menopause: menopause that occurs before age 40

Postmenopause: all the years beyond menopause

Source: North American Menopause Society

We also still don't know all that much about menopause, although we're finding out more all the time. Part of the reason for this lack of knowledge is that modern medicine has traditionally focused its efforts on treating ailments that pertain more to men than to women.

Only during the last 30 years or so has the medical community shown any great interest in women's issues at all, and in menopause in particular. A primary reason for this interest is the sheer number of women who are or will soon be experiencing menopause. Currently, an estimated 40 million American women are in some stage of menopause. This number will increase dramatically in the years ahead as the baby-boom generation continues to age. It is estimated that by the year 2015 almost 50% of the female population will be menopausal.

Another reason behind the lack of information about menopause is that it simply wasn't much of a concern until fairly recently. Until the last 50 years or so, the physical and emotional changes that we now know are part of menopause were simply chalked up as being part of getting older. While women might occasionally attribute a physical woe or a blue feeling to "going through the change," what they went through during this stage in their lives was hardly seen as something that warranted a therapeutic approach. If a woman did seek medical care for some reason, her condition was treated as a disease, not as a normal stage of the aging process.

Prior to the 20th century, many women simply didn't outlive their supplies of their sexual hormones; as a result, problems related to their loss weren't common. As recently as the 1900s, the life expectancy for women in the United States was between 45 and 55. It wasn't until the 1930s that it increased to about age 65. Today, according to the National Center for Health Statistics, the life expectancy for a woman in the United States is 79.8 years (2001 figure). Women who enjoy good health can reasonably expect to live well into their 80s and even their 90s. (Japanese women, by the way, live the longest, with their life expectancy measured at 84.62 years in 2000.)

While life-expectancy rates have increased, the average age for the onset of menopause—between ages 45 and 55—has remained virtually unchanged. This means that most women will spend almost half their lives in one menopausal stage or another, and they'll spend at least one-third of their lives in post-menopause.

Today we know that some of the changes that women go through when they reach middle age are indeed related to menopause, while others are more correctly attributed to the aging process in general. Still, it can be difficult to differentiate which of these changes are directly caused by menopause and which are not. Some may be related to conditions such as diabetes, obesity, hypertension, and thyroid disorders, all of which often develop in both women and men during midlife. Or other hormonal imbalances may be causing symptoms and going completely undetected. For example, as we age, DHEA and growth-hormone levels decline as cortisol and insulin levels tend to elevate providing the person does not have extreme adrenal insufficiency or diabetes. These imbalances often mimic or aggravate the signs and symptoms of menopause.

With the dividing lines between these conditions being as fuzzy or as hidden as they are, it's clear that there are strong connections between those that are related to menopause and those that are not. There is thus a strong case for taking a "whole-body" approach when dealing with all of them.

Sadly, this approach is one that women often have to design for themselves. While menopause is being seen more for what it is— a natural physiological process that all women go through, rather than a disease that leaves women less healthy, less youthful and less womanly—physicians are still woefully uninformed about it and are often ill-equipped to help women navigate this important time of their lives.

If assistance is offered at all, it is generally in the form of hormone replacement therapy—usually based on commonly accepted dosages and rarely customized to meet individual needs. Menopause is as individual as a fingerprint. No two women will experience it in the same way. Yet, most women are subjected to a "one size fits all" approach to menopause treatment. That is, if they receive any treatment at all.

Why Menopause Happens

Once considered a physical disorder caused by hormone deficiencies, menopause is in fact a part of the female reproductive system's natural biological process—a process that begins at birth and continues through each woman's lifetime.

All women are born with a certain number of eggs, which the reproductive hormones—estrogen, progesterone, follicle-stimulating hormone (FSH), and luteinizing hormone (LH)—cause to be released from the ovaries on a fairly regular schedule during the childbearing years. These four hormones, along with other reproductive hormones, work with one another to both regulate ovulation and help maintain pregnancy. Their levels fluctuate throughout each menstrual cycle—at the beginning of the cycle, for example, estrogen levels are high and progesterone levels are low.

At the beginning of a menstrual cycle, follicle-stimulating hormone (FSH) is secreted by the pituitary gland. Located in the brain, this gland controls the entire hormone or endocrine system. FSH, in turn, stimulates the ovaries to produce estrogen hormones.

The level of estrogen continues to rise until it reaches a certain point, at which time the pituitary gland secretes luteinizing hormone (LH). It is this hormone that triggers ovulation at the middle of the menstrual cycle. After the ovaries have released an egg, they then secrete the hormone progesterone—which prevents another egg from being released during this cycle. If the egg isn't fer-

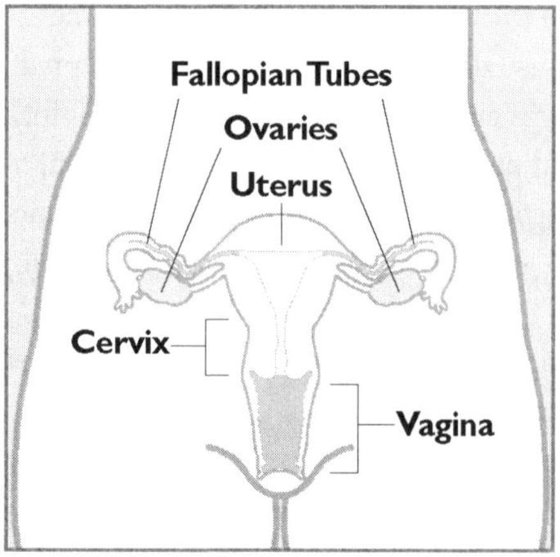

> Estrogen is often referred to as a singular hormone, but it actually consists of three hormones and their metabolites (substances that are either involved in or are byproducts of the metabolism of these hormones) that are grouped together by their similar qualities.

Fallopian Tubes
Ovaries
Uterus
Cervix
Vagina

Figure 1: Female Anatomy

tilized, the uterus sheds its lining causing a period. At the same time, there is a dramatic and rapid fall in estrogen and progesterone levels and the whole process begins again. If the egg is fertilized, it is implanted into the wall of the uterus for development.

Natural menopause—that is, menopause that is not surgically induced or caused by an injury to the ovaries—usually begins sometime in a woman's late 40s, when the ovaries start making less estrogen and progesterone. As the production of these hormones slows, periods become irregular. Ovulation becomes less likely, although periods can and still do take place as a result of high levels of FSH and LH in the bloodstream. In fact, one of the basic screening tests for menopause measures the level of FSH in the blood. A high level indicates that you are menopausal.

As production of the reproductive hormones diminishes, the time between menstrual cycles increases until menstruation comes to an end. This process is different for every woman. Some women go through a period of several years during which hormone levels fluctuate wildly and wreak havoc with their menstrual cycles, causing them to get shorter or longer and heavier or lighter.

One period might be significantly heavier than usual, with an almost frightening flood of dark, clotted blood that no amount of protection can entirely contain; this heavy period might be followed by several periods during which discharge is normal or light, or there may be no period at all for several months. Other women experience a more gradual decline in hormone levels and simply stop menstruating one day.

According to researchers, 15 percent of women have absolutely no problem with menopause, 15 percent experience severe problems, and the rest fall somewhere in-between.

When Menopause Happens

Menopause generally doesn't take place at a constant rate, nor does it follow the same timeline in every woman. Women can experience naturally occurring menopause as early as age 40 and as late as age 58 (in the Western world, the average age of menopause is 51), which means that chronological age is not a good indication of when a woman can expect menstruation to come to an end.

Factors Affecting the Onset of Menopause

Researchers have identified two key factors that can influence when menopause actually takes place. First, women who smoke have been found to experience menopause approximately 1 ½ to two years earlier than those who don't. It is believed that smoking causes a decrease in the level of estrogens secreted by the ovaries. How long a woman smokes and how many cigarettes she smokes during that period were also found to influence the onset of menopause.

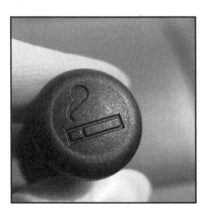

Genetics also plays a role in determining when menopause begins. If your mother went through natural menopause, the age at which she did can be a good indication of when you will.

The following factors might also be related to an earlier than average onset of menopause:

▶ not having children

▶ having medically treated depression

▶ suffering from poor nutrition

▶ being exposed to toxic chemicals

▶ having undergone pelvic radiation to treat childhood cancer

▶ having had epilepsy, especially for women who have had frequent seizures

Later than average onset of menopause is believed to be related to the following:

▶ more than one pregnancy

▶ fibroids

▶ higher body-mass-index levels

▶ higher cognitive scores in childhood

▶ premenstrual syndrome

Such factors as use of oral contraceptives, the age at which menstruation began, socioeconomic or marital status, and race have not been found to affect the age at which menopause begins.

The Stages of Menopause

As previously mentioned, changes in the menstrual cycle are often the first indications that a woman is entering into perimenopause, the transitional time that precedes menopause. Hot flashes are another early indication, and may begin when women are still menstruating regularly. The hormonal roller coaster can begin when one is as young as 35 or 40 and is especially problematic for women with histories of female hormone imbalances, which can cause such problems as PMS, endometriosis, and ovarian cysts.

The median age for the onset of the menopausal transition is 47.5 years. For most women, the transition lasts approximately four years. Only about 10 percent of women cease menstruating abruptly, experiencing no menstrual irregularity.

Perimenopause is also marked by other hormone-driven symptoms, including the following:

- mood swings
- irritability
- problems remembering things; feeling "foggy"
- sleep disruptions
- vaginal dryness
- depression
- general aches and pains that can't be attributed to anything else

In 2001, the Stages of Reproductive Aging Workshop (STRAW), sponsored by the North American Menopause Society (NAMS), the National Institutes of Health, the American Society for Reproductive Medicine, and the National Institute of Child Health and Human Development, developed a reproductive-aging timeline that illustrates the stages that a woman's reproductive system goes through. It divides the reproductive-aging process into seven stages, with five stages preceding and two following the final menstrual period. You can easily find the chart online on a number of different websites.

As noted by STRAW, however, this timeline should be considered a *general* road map to reproductive aging, as many healthy women won't follow the pattern exactly. Some will fluctuate between stages, or skip a stage entirely.

Health Risks Associated With Menopause

Of deep concern to women going through menopause are the health risks associated with declining hormone levels. HRT helps preserve bone density, protecting women from potentially debilitating and even fatal bone fractures. The loss of estrogen in the body leaves women significantly more susceptible to heart disease, strokes, blood clots, and osteoporosis. For this reason, a number of experts still believe that combination HRT is appropriate for diminishing the large drop in bone density that occurs right after menopause.

Heart disease is the No. 1 killer of American women. For long-term heart protection during menopause, women should consider all the options, including for example, drugs that lower cholesterol and blood-pressure levels, healthy eating, exercise, and weight control.

Osteoporosis is another important health issue for middle-aged women. The risk of developing it increases as you age. There are also a number of factors that contribute to it, including the following:

▶ smoking

▶ heavy use of alcohol

▶ a family history of osteoporosis

▶ surgical removal of the ovaries as well as radiation therapy for ovarian cancer

▶ long-term use of steroid drugs, such as cortisone

▶ poor nutrition overall—inadequate calories, protein, or essential fats

▶ calcium deficiencies and using poorly absorbable forms of calcium

▶ magnesium deficiencies and challenges with absorption of magnesium, which can function as a laxative

▶ vitamin-D deficiencies

▶ hypochlorhydria—levels of HCL in the stomach that are inadequate to begin the process of absorbing calcium

▶ trace mineral deficiencies, including a deficiency of boron or strontium

▶ a lack of exercise

While it has been shown to be beneficial in addressing one's risk of osteoporosis, HRT isn't the only answer. Improving one's diet, doing weight-bearing exercises, getting all 90 essential nutrients (amino acids, fatty acids, vitamins, minerals, and trace minerals), and taking medications designed to improve bone mass are other proven approaches to slowing the rate of bone loss that can take place as estrogen levels drop.

On the Other Side of Menopause

Menopause is, without question, a life-changing experience. It affects each woman differently, and each woman approaches it in a different way. Many women feel a certain sense of loss as they leave their childbearing years behind. If their identities have largely been shaped by their roles as wives and mothers and they're facing other emotional upheavals at the same time, such as seeing children leave for college and experiencing other changes at home, the loss can be overwhelming. Depression and other emotional problems are not uncommon among peri-menopausal women.

Other women welcome the positives that menopause brings to their lives. Worrying about contraception is a thing of the past; so too are the pressures of raising a young family, establishing a career, and dealing with the demands on one's time that these responsibilities require.

The postmenopausal years can be, and often are, some of the most fulfilling, productive, and creative years in a woman's life. No longer having to be as focused on the needs of others, and being able to focus on one's own self-expression, can be extremely uplifting and freeing. The fact that postmenopausal women have lower levels of clinical depression than any other group is indicative of how truly wonderful the second half of a woman's life can be.

Because each woman experiences menopause differently, there is no way to predict what menopause will be like for you. However, meeting menopause head on, and taking a proactive approach by addressing its symptoms and discomforts, can put you in good stead for the easiest transit possible through the menopausal years.

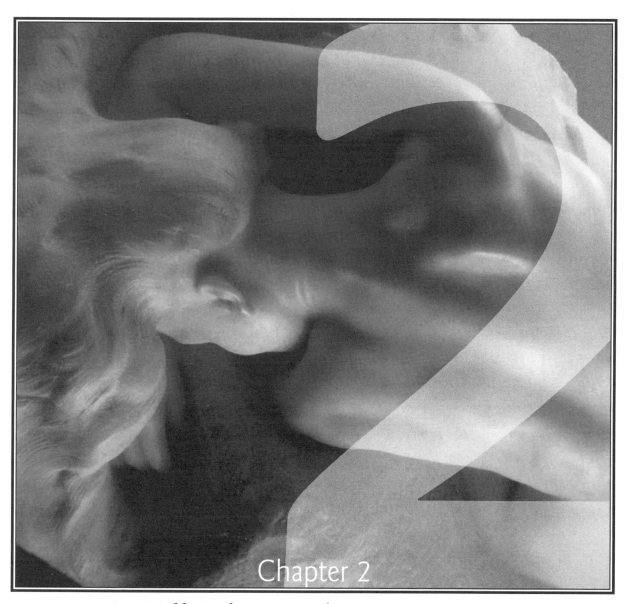

Chapter 2

It's All About the Hormones

Chapter 2
It's All About the Hormones

Taking a proactive approach begins with really understanding the role that hormones play both in menopause and in life in general. It's hard to overstate the importance of hormones in the functioning of the body, yet their importance is seldom stressed by the mainstream. As a result most of us know very little about them.

Some of the following material is very basic. Some of it is a bit more difficult. All of it however is very important to the understanding of what happens to the female body during menopause and is well worth reading.

Exactly What Are Hormones?

To begin with, hormones are either chemical substances produced by cells located in various glands in the body that affect the activities of other cells or laboratory-created substances that are designed to mimic the action of naturally produced hormones. Hormones function as chemical messengers sending specific instructions that activate a whole range of responses in target cells and in the nuclei of cells. People, other animals, and plants all manufacture hormones, which are carried throughout their systems in body fluid or in sap. In this chapter, we'll primarily discuss the hormones found in humans.

As part of the complex machine that is the human body, hormones are the substances that maintain proper functioning and balance. Without hormones, we would die. It's as simple as that. But this is where simplicity ends. In fact, while we today know a great deal about hormones and their functions, there is quite a bit that is yet to be discovered about the complex actions and interactions of these vital substances, and that remains a continuing challenge for researchers in the quest to unlock the body's secrets.

What we do know is that within each hormone is a specific set of instructions that is designed to tell certain cells what to do. Once hormones reach their targeted destinations, they will, depending on what these instructions are, do one of three things:

▸ direct cell function

▸ activate cell function

▸ control cell function

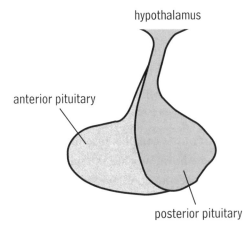

Figure 2: The Pituitary Gland

Hormones fall into three chemical classes—peptides, proteins, and steroids. They are all produced by glands in the body's endocrine system. Major glands in this system include the hypothalamus, the pituitary, the pineal gland, the adrenal glands, the thyroid and parathyroid glands, the pancreas, the testes, and the ovaries. Of these, the pituitary is often referred to as the "master gland." That's because it releases many hormones that affect the release of others.

To help them receive their information from hormones, cells have receptor sites. There are two different types of sites: membrane receptors, which are located on cell surfaces, and nucleus, or cytoplasm receptors, which are inside of cells. Hormones that trigger chemical reactions via membrane receptors act much more rapidly than those that work inside cells. The latter hormones, which affect cell DNA and direct the manufacturing of specific enzymes and proteins, by nature act more slowly and are in the class of hormones known as steroids.

When a circulating hormone reaches its target cell, it slides into these receptor sites similar to how a key fits into a lock or how interlocking puzzle pieces fit together. Because the actions that hormones govern are so complex and so individual, the receptor sites and the hormones that fit into them are designed to be a perfect fit for each other. Some hormones are chemically very similar and might be able to fit into receptor sites meant for other hormones, but they either won't be able to do anything while they're there or at least won't work as well. In the case of steroid hormones that are not molecularly identical, this partial fit can, however, lead to incorrect information being transmitted to nuclear DNA, causing abnormal cell function, cell activation, or cell control.

Hormones have three basic functions inside the human body. They control growth, energy production, and storage; water and salt metabolism; and sexual and reproductive actions. Once hormones complete their work, they are either broken down and deactivated by their target cells or continue their passage through the bloodstream to the liver to be metabolized. They can then be made into new hormones. If they're not, they are excreted.

Hormones are either stored in the glands that make them or immediately released into the bloodstream as soon as they're made. Finally, hormones work synergistically in so-called feedback loops designed to keep hor-

mone levels in balance. The most common type of feedback loop is negative, but in some cases positive feedback loops can also control hormone release.

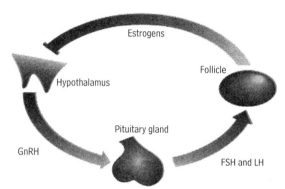

Figure 3: Typical Negative Feedback Loop
(Diagram courtesy of Dr. John Kimball, Kimball's Biology Pages.)

This checks-and-balances system is a key characteristic of the endocrine system. When hormone levels are tested, it is to determine how well this system is working and to detect any problems in the delicate balances between various hormones.

Different Functions for Different Hormones

While we often think of the sex hormones —estrogen, progesterone, and testosterone—

Major Endocrine Glands

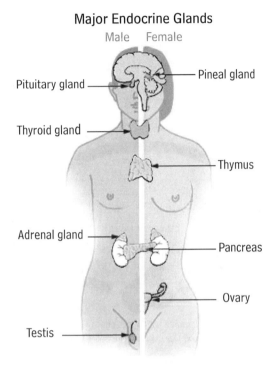

Male   Female

Pituitary gland ——

Pineal gland

Thyroid gland ——

Thymus

Adrenal gland ——

Pancreas

Ovary

Testis ——

Figure 4: Major Endocrine Glands

whenever hormones are discussed, the body produces many other hormones in addition to these. The ones that follow are the most important when it comes to understanding the role that these chemical messengers play during menopause. As you read through the descriptions, pay particular attention to the interactions between various hormone groups.

For ease of explanation, I'll organize the following discussion by gland, starting with the "master gland," the pituitary.

Pituitary Hormones

A pea-sized structure that lies at the base of the brain, the pituitary gland (see Figure 2) has three parts, one of which, the anterior, is of most interest to our discussion. It is controlled by the hypothalamus.

Anterior pituitary: The anterior pituitary secretes six peptide hormones of concern for

menopausal women: corticotropin (ACTH), thyroid-stimulating hormone (TSH), follicle-stimulating hormone (FSH), luteinizing hormone (LH), growth hormone (GH), and prolactin. With the exception of growth hormone, all anterior pituitary hormones regulate the activity of other glands. Growth hormone affects all cells of the body.

Corticotropin (ACTH)	It stimulates the production and release of adrenal steroids and is regulated by cortisol levels in the blood, individual biorhythms, and stress.
Follicle-stimulating hormone (FSH)	It targets the testes in men and the ovaries in women. In the testes it facilitates the making of sperm. In the ovaries it stimulates the growth and development of the follicle. It also stimulates testosterone production in men and estrogen and progesterone production in women. Release of FSH is regulated by a negative feedback system (see Figure 3) that incorporates these hormones. When women become menopausal, FSH rises attempting to stimulate ovarian production of estrogen and progesterone without an ovarian response.
Thyroid-stimulating Hormone (TSH)	As its name implies, TSH stimulates the synthesis and secretion of thyroid hormones. It is controlled by feedback from those hormones. The more thyroid hormones are produced, the less TSH is released (a negative feedback loop) and vice versa.
Luteinizing-hormone (LH)	Another hormone that targets the sex organs, luteinizing hormone triggers testosterone production in men. In women, it targets ovarian follicles, telling them, in effect, to secrete estrogen in the first half of the menstrual cycle. It also triggers ovulation and tells the now-empty follicle to develop into a corpus luteum, which secretes progesterone during the latter part of the menstrual cycle.
Growth-hormone (GH)	GH oversees the entire process of normal body growth by binding to receptors on the surface of the cells of the liver and stimulating them to release growth factor-1 (IGF-1), an insulin-type hormone that promotes bone and cartilage growth; RNA formation; protein, fat, and glucose metabolism; and electrolyte balance. GH levels tend to decline

with age, and many menopausal women are GH and IGF-1 deficient. As a result, they may experience weight gain, a low libido, reduced endurance, excessively thin or wrinkled skin, hair loss, depression, impaired concentration, and insomnia.

Prolactin

The anterior pituitary gland also produces prolactin, which stimulates breast development and lactation after childbirth. Excess prolactin can cause amenorrhea, infertility, and galactorrhea (milk discharge from the breasts). Significant prolactin release inhibits ovarian production of hormones. Although large amounts of prolactin are produced in pregnancy, they are counteracted by the large amounts of estrogen, progesterone, and other steroids produced by the placenta during pregnancy. Nonlactating women can overproduce prolactin to the point of ovarian suppression and amenorrhea. This may be due to hypothyroidism, use of birth control pills (which are high in synthetic estrogens), and chronic stress, with high cortisol release causing more release of prolactin or high serotonin because of SSRI drugs prescribed for depression.

Adrenal Hormones

The adrenal glands are two small, triangular structures that are loosely attached to the kidneys. They have two separate parts: The outer layer, or adrenal cortex, surrounds the other part, the adrenal medulla. The cells of the adrenal cortex secrete a variety of steroid hormones. These hormones are not stored but rather synthesized and released as needed.

Prior to puberty, all of the body's steroidal sex hormones are manufactured by the adrenal glands. After puberty, the adrenal glands share this responsibility with the body's sex glands—the testes and the ovaries.

Steroid hormones have the unique characteristic of carrying their hormonal messages past the cell membrane and cytoplasm to the

DNA of the nucleus of the cell. There are additional hormones and even vitamins, which, while not classified as steroids, act similarly in influencing cell nuclear DNA. They include thyroid hormone, vitamin A, and vitamin D. The steroids made in the adrenal cortex include DHEA, cortisol, aldosterone, androstenedione, testosterone, progesterone, and estrogen with the last four being produced in the ovaries and testicles as well.

Steroids, by interacting directly with genetic programming via nuclear DNA, help to determine which genes are turned on or turned off. These genes then determine which proteins are manufactured for a variety of purposes. One of the most fascinating purposes is the manufacturing of proteins used to biosynthesize the receptor sites on cells, as well as receptor sites on the cell nucleus used for hormone-receptor binding. Receptor sites increase and decrease as demand changes. The more circulating hormone available, the more receptors are biosynthesized and vice versa. In a sense, the creative force of the universe is telling us that these steroid hormones are powerful intracellular communicators. This is all the more reason to use biologically identical molecules of hormone replacement as medication, if such replacement therapy is used at all.

Adrenal-cortex hormones fall into three classes, as seen below. The secretion of ACTH by the pituitary gland triggers them all.

Aldosterone	It regulates potassium, magnesium, and sodium levels in body fluids and tells the kidneys to retain sodium and water to maintain normal blood pressure. Excess potassium intake relative to sodium intake increases aldosterone production. As aldosterone production goes up, it activates DNA in the adrenals and ovaries/testicles to increase production of steroid hormones. Aldosterone production determines the rate of all other adrenal-steroid production. Aldosterone, by its enzyme activation, controls the rate-limiting step of the biosynthesis of steroid hormones, which is the conversion of cholesterol into pregnenalone. Therefore, the common use of ACE inhibitors that lower aldosterone ends up lowering adrenal-steroid production overall. Aldosterone also increases the cardiac and brain ionic-cell charge.

Androgens (DHEA, testosterone)

They enhance one' sex drive and produce mild male features in women. Such as facial hair, and a more male-type body shape. (They are also produced in the ovaries and testicles.) DHEA is the main androgen produced in the adrenals and is the major body steroid. In fact, there is more DHEA in the body then any other androgen. It is an anabolic steroid that builds up one's body form and muscle mass, though to a lesser extent than does testosterone. DHEA has a higher concentration than does any other steroid in the blood vessels. It serves as the base substance for the synthesis of both testosterone and estradiol prior to puberty. Women, however, must depend on the adrenal cortex for the continuing synthesis of the majority of their androgen hormones. Women's bodies also convert some androgen into estrone to compensate for the loss of ovarian estrogen after menopause. In men, after puberty, the testes take over testosterone production. DHEA levels increase from age 7 to about age 25. Levels then gradually decline to a level of about 10% of peak adolescent production in the last years of life. DHEA has been implicated as a rejuvenation and antiaging hormone by many authors. DHEA levels tend to antagonize cortisol production. As DHEA levels decline with aging, cortisol tends to increase. With this increase of cortisol comes an increase of insulin and a tendency toward central weight gain. Insulin and cortisol are the two most fat-cell-stimulating hormones.

Testosterone

Testosterone is made in the ovaries and adrenals in both sexes. After menopause, when ovarian testosterone production falls, a healthy adrenal gland takes over as the sole source of testosterone in women. Testosterone is an anabolic steroid like DHEA but more potent in its effects. Testosterone converts into dihydrotestosterone (DHT), which is a 10 times more potent anabolic steroid than testosterone. While testosterone can convert into estrogen, DHT cannot.

Fat cells contain an aromatoase enzyme that converts testosterone into estrogen. The more fat is present, the more testosterone will be converted to estrogen. Also, the presence of zinc inhibits the enzyme conversion of testosterone into estrogen. You may also be deficient in methyl groups from a lack of dietary methionine. When testosterone loses its methyl group, it becomes estradiol. (See Figure 5 below.)

When testosterone loses its methyl group it becomes estradiol.

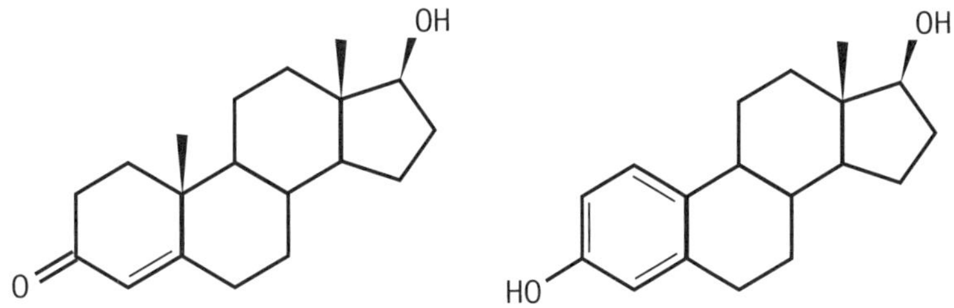

Figure 5: Testosterone and Estradiol

Testosterone, as a potent anabolic steroid, binds to nuclear DNA, sending a clear message to build strength, muscle mass, and bone mass and to produce general rejuvenation. Low testosterone, on the other hand, increases wear and tear, degeneration, and the aging process. With testosterone, as with anything else, you can get too much of a good thing, resulting in excessive facial hair, acne, and a host of other symptoms and complications.

Women undergoing menopause may experience such symptoms as a low libido, hair loss, reduced muscle mass, increased fat, and increased "wear and tear" due to a drop in testosterone. This drop in testosterone, while not uncommon, is often ignored and not tested for by physicians prescribing HRT.

Cortisol

Responsible for many metabolic activities in the body, including balancing of blood-sugar levels, cortisol also reduces inflammation and suppresses immune responses. A body under stress produces higher amounts of cortisol. This shifts the body's work from cell maintenance to cell survival. As cortisol is released, extra blood sugar is released to meet the physical demand of stress. Exercising muscles will use the extra sugar, and there is no need for insulin release. In the case of mental stress, however, the excess sugar is still produced, and since the muscles aren't reacting, the sugar has nowhere to go. Excess insulin is produced, and in this sense chronic nonphysical (mental and emotional) stress can contribute to obesity because of a lack of physical activity and because of an increased production of insulin in response to high blood-sugar levels. As cortisol levels rise, insulin's effects are enhanced. Insulin is the main fat-inducing hormone, followed by cortisol. Weight gain as you age is often, at least in part, due to elevations in insulin and cortisol.

As cortisol levels rise, DHEA levels decline and vice versa. Cortisol is a catabolic steroid that consumes body-structure and fuel needs instead of building muscle mass in the way that DHEA and testosterone (anabolic steroids) do. Taking cortisol for prolonged periods causes a loss of muscle mass, along with a gain in fat and fluid retention. Instead of producing rejuvenating effects like those produced by DHEA, catabolic steroids like cortisol manage survival activities, inflammation control, and responses to stress. As an example, healthy joints need cortisol to stay lubricated and avoid inflammation. Cortisol binds to receptors on joint cells, reducing inflammation.

Cortisol also has a direct effect on the production of androgens. Excess cortisol release causes the ovaries and testicles to release androgens (testosterone, androstenedione, and DHEA). If, however, cortisol remains elevated, this gradually lowers DHEA levels. It is common for men and women in midlife to have high cortisol and low DHEA levels while suffering with obesity and stress maladaption.

Adrenaline and Noradreneline

The adrenal medulla is part of the body's nervous system. It contains masses of neurons that produce the neurotransmitters noradrenaline (or norepinephrine / NE) and adrenaline (or epinephrine/EP), which are hormones that govern the actions of neurons or muscle fibers. They are both triggered in response to physical or mental stress.

Noradrenaline and adrenaline might be familiar to you as the "fight or flight" hormones. They prepare the body for immediate action by increasing heart and metabolic rates. Both are released by the adrenal medulla in response to stress.

Epinephrine

Epinephrine is a hormone that plays an integral role in the body's physiological stress response to conditions that are physically threatening to the body. The hormone is secreted by the adrenal medulla. When it is released into the bloodstream, epinephrine binds to multiple receptors and has numerous effects throughout the body.

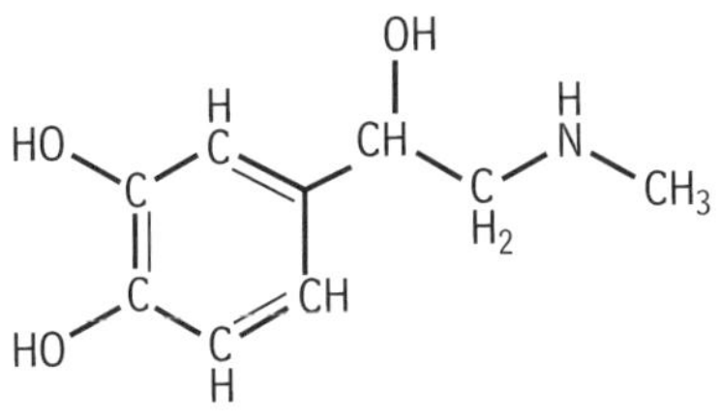

Figure 6: Epinephrine

▸ It constricts peripheral blood vessels and increases blood supply to the heart, muscles, and liver. Since the muscle or liver mass is so large, the net effect of epinephrine is to lower blood-vessel resistance, and thereby control high blood pressure.

▸ It increases blood sugar by stimulating the liver to break down stored glycogen.

▸ It dilates the bronchi and the pupils.

▸ It reduces the clotting time of blood.

▸ It causes the hair to stand on end.

Norepinephrine

Norepinephrine is a hormone that is both released into the blood from the adrenal glands and released into the nervous system as a neurotransmitter. It is one of the "stress hormones" and it has a number of effects on the body.

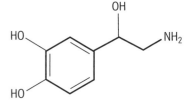

Figure 7: Norepinephrine

▸ It strongly constricts blood vessels.

▸ It raises blood pressure.

▸ It converts into epinephrine with the cofactor SAMe (s-adenosyl methionine). SAMe donates its one methyl group to turn norepinephrine into epinephrine. If you are methyl-donor deficient (due to a diet low in methionine or high in homocysteine, which reduces the recycling of methionine), this deficiency can make norepinephrine accumulate in the body. Since norepinephrine has potent vasoconstrictive properties, this, in turn, can lead to hypertension or cause existing hypertension to worsen. Some newer drugs used for attention deficit disorder can also increase norepinephrine and can cause high blood pressure as a side effect.

Under normal circumstances, the adrenal medulla secretes approximately 90% epinephrine and only 10% norepinephrine. Only when adequate cortisol is present can the cell receptors optimally recognize epinephrine and norepinephrine message content. Noradrenaline and adrenaline also cause increased ACTH secretions. So, as you can see, maintaining a balance between and among all the hormones is essential.

Ovarian Hormones

Steroid hormones are also produced by the ovaries (and by the testes in men). The ovaries secrete three different types of hormones—estrogens, progesterone, and testosterone. As steroids, all of these hormones can enter freely into cells, their nuclei, and DNA programing , which is why they affect so many of the body's systems.

Estrogens

There are actually three estrogens—estrone/E1, estradiol/E2, and estriol/E3. Of these, estradiol is the most potent and estriol is the most abundant. Estradiol also converts into estrone, which is thought to be the form of estrogen that causes breast cancer if it is metabolized into excessive amounts of 4-or 16-hydroxy estrone.

Premarin, made from horse estrogen and estrone sulphate, is converted primarily into estrone in the intestinal tract. Horse mares' urine also contains alpha-estradiol, which does not naturally occur in women. Alpha-estradiol is 30 times more potent than estradiol. Additionally, Premarin also contains potent horse equilins not found in humans.

In the body, as you can see in the tables below, estrone (E1) converts into estradiol (E2) and estradiol converts back to estrone, as well as estriol (E3). E1 is then converted into 2 (the safest and most protective metabolite), 4 (the most potent free radical, causing cell damage and increasing cancer risks), or 16 (the most carcinogenic hydroxyestrone.) Depending upon the individual, she will convert E1 and E2 into more or less of the safer two.

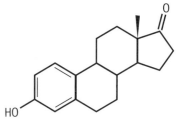

Figure 8: Estrone

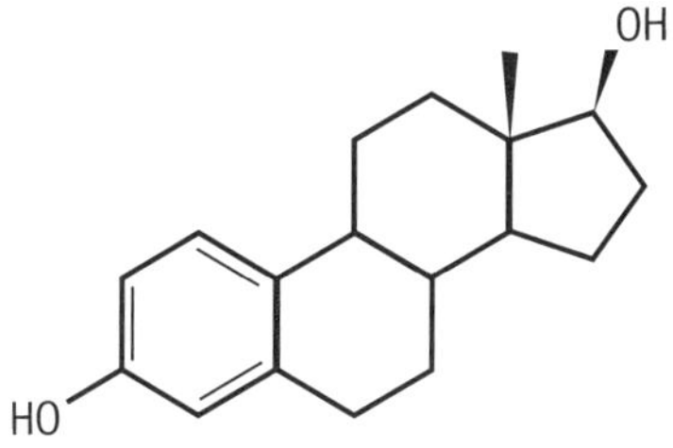

Figure 9: Estradiol

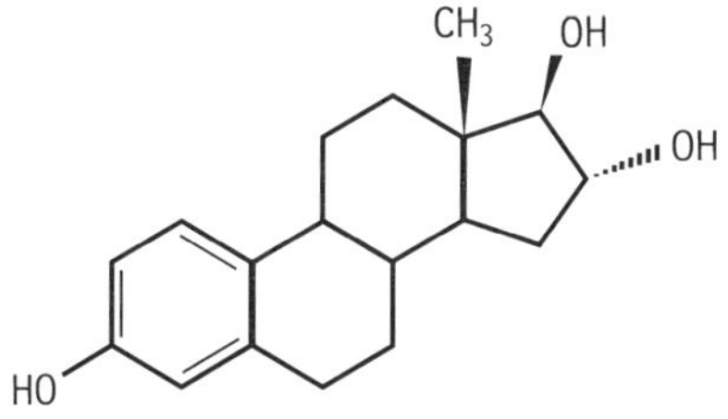

Figure 10: Estriol

Table 1: Estrogen Conversion

Hormone	Estrone	Estradiol	Estriol
Abbreviation	E1 ⟷	E2 ⟶	E3
Relative Potency	12X	80X	1X
Approx. % in Body	10-20%	10-20%	60-80%

Table 2: Estrogen Conversion

Hormone	Estrone	Estradiol	Estriol
Abbreviation	E1 ⟷	E2 ⟶	E3
Hydroxyestrone*	2	4	16

* Note that 2 is protective, 4 and 16 are carcinogenic.

Table 3: Prescription Forms of Estrogen

ESTROGEN TYPE	Rx. SOURCES	POTENCY & CARCINOGENICITY
Estradiol (E2) 80X	• Estraderm patch (0.05 & 0.01) • Estrace (all estradiol) tablets and cream • Premarin tablets & cream conjugated estrogen, estradiol and estrone from pregnant horse mare's urine • Compounded natural estradiol from wild yam or soybean	• Half life 16-18 hours • Most potent, most carcinogenic
Estrone (E1) 12X	• Ortho-est or Ogen (piperazine estrone sulfate) tablets (0.625 & 1.25) • Ogen vaginal cream (1.5 mg/gram = 1/4 tsp.) • Estratest & estratest HS (esterified estrogens, principally estrone) 0.625/1.25 mg estrone, 1.25/2.5 mg methytestosterone. 3 weeks on, one week off • Compounded natural estrone from wild yam or soybean	• 12 hours • In-between in potency and carcinogenicity
Estriol (E3) 1X	• Compounded natural estriol derived from soybeans, and/or yams	• Half life 6-8 hours • Least potent, least carcinogenic • Cancer protective in several studies

Estrogens, as I am sure you are already aware, play a key role in menstruation and pregnancy and are responsible for producing secondary sex characteristics in women. Estrogens are produced in the highest amount in the first half of the menstrual cycle. They are responsible for the building up of the endometrial lining of the uterus throughout the menstrual cycle. If estrogen excess occurs, a woman can develop endometrial hyperplasia (an excessive buildup in the endometrium) or breakthrough bleeding in the middle of her cycle. This estrogen dominance can occur indirectly from a relative progesterone deficiency as well. Estrogens can also negate the actions of parathyroid hormone (see below), helping to minimize calcium loss from bones. Estrogens also promote blood clotting. Many individuals with either estrogen dominance or a prior history of birth-control-pill use may have a low-grade chronic-coagulation disorder that remains hidden and undiagnosed. This places these individuals at a greater risk for cardiovascular disease. Testing your fibrinogen levels and bleeding times for platelet aggregation can help identify if you have this problem. Treatments like essential fatty acids, aspirin, and Nattokinase can be helpful as part of a total plan to thin your blood naturally and safely.

The Role of Estrogen

- prepares the uterine lining for pregnancy
- stimulates breast tissue growth for lactation
- supports mental well being
- promotes bone health
- promotes and supports vaginal health

Estrogen dominance can occur from exposure to what are known as estrogen mimickers, chemicals introduced into the environment that mimic hormones. This dominance can also occur from prolonged use of synthetic progesterone. Synthetic hormone replacement and birth-control-pills can cause further estrogen dominance.

Excess insulin caused by insulin resistance increases the conversion of various hormones to estradiol, resulting in an increased estrogen pool. Aromatase enzyme activity in various tissues, especially fat (andipose) tissue, increases the conversion of androstenedione to estrone, further aggravating any tendencies toward excess estrogen (estrogen dominance). So, in general, women who are both insulin resistant (pre-diabetic) and overweight are often in need of hormone balancing. Sex hormone binding globulin (SHBG) is responsible for binding sex hormones like estrogen and then gradually releasing these hormones into the circulation. Low levels of SHBG increase the amount of free estrogen circulating contributing to estrogen dominance. See the resource section for information on a laboratory I recommend for doing a comprehensive women's health panel with SHBG levels.

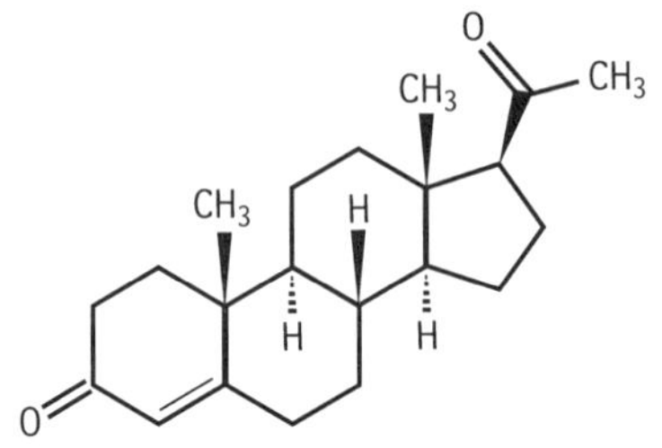

Figure 11: Progesterone

Progesterone:

Progesterone is responsible for many metabolic actions in the body. It also helps maintain pregnancy, affects insulin levels, slows down the transit of food through the intestines, regulates blood pressure, and can contribute to sweet cravings in women who suffer from premenstrual syndrome. Progesterone binds to receptors on osteoblasts (bone-building cells), which increases the rate of bone formation and remodeling. High levels may cause depression. LH triggers progesterone. In times of stress, the body converts progesterone into adrenal hormones, which can cause elevated estrogen levels, as there's not enough progesterone to regulate them. Women who have had a hysterectomy and oophorectomy are given estrogens without progesterone, forcing their adrenal glands to take up the slack and manufacture as much progesterone as possible. This often causes estrogen-replacement-induced adrenal exhaustion and stress, leading to DHEA depletion and if unchecked ultimately cortisone depletion as well (adrenal insufficiency/adrenal failure).

Testosterone:

Testosterone is the primary male sex hormone. In men, it's essential for producing sperm. In women, testosterone boosts their libido and energy, helps to maintain muscle mass, strengthens bone, and heightens response to sexual stimulation.

Thyroid Hormones:

A double-lobed structure located in the neck, the thyroid gland synthesizes and secretes thyroxin, also known as T4; triiodothyronine also known as T3; and calcitonin. T3, which is the active form of thyroid hormone, is also metabolized from T4 in the liver and other tissues.

The thyroid is home to the parathyroid gland, which consists of four tiny structures embedded in the rear surface of the thyroid gland. The parathyroid secretes PTH, which increases blood calcium.

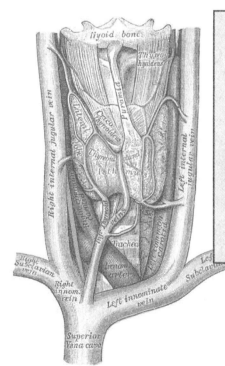

Seventy-five percent of the hormones made by the thyroid is T4 or thyroxin; 25 percent is T3 or triiodothyronine. By using an enzyme called 5' deiodinase, which removes one atom of iodine from T4, the liver and other tissues convert T4 into T3, the active form of the hormone. This requires selenium as a cofactor. More than 80 percent of circulating T3 is made in this way rather than by the thyroid gland.

Figure 12: Thyroid Gland

Thyroxine (T4) along with the active form triiodothyronine (T3):	It stimulates your body's metabolism by increasing cell-energy release and increases heart rate, heat production, and brain activity. T4 and T3 production are stimulated by TSH.
Calcitonin:	It lowers blood-calcium levels by causing calcium retention in bone.
Parathyroid Hormone (PTH):	It increases blood calcium levels by stimulating bone breakdown and calcium release.

It should be clear by now that many hormones are affected by other hormones, or affect them. It therefore follows that when the balance of one is thrown off, it can trigger a chain reaction in the body that affects the way in which a number of systems function. Or, as Deepak Chopra puts it, "Touch one strand and the whole web trembles."

Synthetic hormones, in particular, can wreak havoc with the body, because they don't work exactly like naturally produced hormones do. Because of their altered function, they disrupt natural hormonal feedback loops—either by remaining in the body too long or by not triggering the correct responses at their receptor sites. When this happens, the adrenal, reproductive, and thyroid systems can't communicate properly and hormone levels become unbalanced. This is why it is so crucial for physicians to prescribe only molecularly identical hormone replacement for their patients.

Other factors that can influence the balance of hormone levels include the following:

▸ diet and nutritional deficiency states

▸ stress

▸ certain drug therapies

Hormones Bound and Unbound

Hormones circulate in the body through the bloodstream. They are either transported by carrier proteins that are specifically designed for this purpose or are free-form.

Peptide and protein-based hormones, which are water-soluble, don't need a carrier to circulate. Steroid hormones, which are synthesized from cholesterol and are therefore fat-based, aren't water-soluble and <u>do need</u> carrier proteins to circulate. The sex hormones are bound with sex-binding globulins. The specific carrier proteins they need are synthesized in the liver.

When hormones are bound to a carrier, they are inactive. Only a small number—between 1 and 5 percent—of steroid hormones are able to break loose from carrier proteins and enter into the bloodstream to their target tissues.

Many factors can affect free hormone levels, causing levels to fluctuate greatly. For example, obesity, hypothyroidism, and insulin levels all can decrease androgen levels. Pregnancy and hyperthyroidism increase estrogen levels. Medications that depend on proteins for transport in the body can compete with hormones for these carrier proteins. This leads to higher levels of free unbound hormones circulating in the body, causing symptoms of hormone excess. Other medications have the opposite effect, causing higher levels of bound hormones and lower levels of free active hormones.

When you treat the symptoms of menopause, it's very important to try to achieve a balance among the ovarian, adrenal, thyroid, and pituitary hormones by assessing their levels early on to develop a baseline against which future tests can be measured. Why test all of these hormones? Because hormonal imbalances can cause certain symptoms or groups of symptoms that can't be fully addressed unless the specific hormones involved are measured. Furthermore, prescribing one hormone can and often does affect others. It's the chain reaction I mentioned earlier. For example, giving DHEA inevitably lowers cortisol levels and vice versa. If DHEA is low, growth hormone may be low and insulin and/or cortisol may be elevated. Giving estrogen can cause a need for more thyroid replacement in a person who is hypothyroid. Hormones do not act in isolation. The levels of any one hormone can affect the levels of other hormones.

During perimenopause, ovarian estrogen, testosterone, and progesterone levels naturally decline; this leads to a strain on the adrenal glands as they attempt to release as much of these hormones as possible. If a woman is under considerable stress, her adrenal-cortisol levels may be high and her DHEA levels low, further impairing her adrenal gland's ability to meet the need for estrogen, testosterone, and progesterone support. If a woman has gradually accumulated excess estrogen throughout her life, this estrogen dominance may have reduced her thyroid-binding and thyroid utilization.

As we age, growth hormone and IGF1 levels decline. Therefore, a common scenario in menopause is low progesterone first followed by low estrogen and then by low testosterone. High cortisol, low DHEA, low growth hormone, and low IGF1 with impaired thyroid metabolism and a history of estrogen dominance will lead to weight gain. Therefore, in order to properly balance hormone replacement in menopause, not only estrogen and progesterone levels but also, but DHEA, testosterone, cortisol, thyroid, IGF1, and insulin levels need to be monitored.

As DHEA levels decline, IGF1 and growth-hormone levels tend to decline as well. Many menopausal women still complain of just not feeling their best (feeling tired, being overweight, having memory problems, etc.) even when they are on optimal customized hormone replacement therapy of natural Triest and progesterone. This occurs because other underlying hormonal imbalances have not been diagnosed or corrected, such as high cortisol, low DHEA, low testosterone, low GH, and low IGF1 associated with insulin resistance and/or dysglycemia and poor thyroid utilization. To make matters worse, many women's diets, even those of women who take supplements, are low in a variety of essential nutrients, including essential amino acids, essential fatty acids, some vitamins, minerals, and trace minerals. These essential nutrients are necessary to synthesize each and every one of the hormones. Without them, the body can't effectively produce the hormones it needs.

One of my most gratifying moments as a physician is seeing menopausal women return feeling better than they have in years as a result of balancing all of these hormones. This is something that is so often overlooked in mainstream approaches. Verifying this balance with lab monitoring is icing on the cake. Getting back a balanced 24-hour urinary hormone panel that also verifies the safe metabolizing of estrogens in balance with progesterone metabolites, testosterone, cortisol, DHEA with normal IGF1, insulin, and thyroid hormone is scientific verification of what a woman is already feeling, and what I as a physician have worked so hard to achieve.

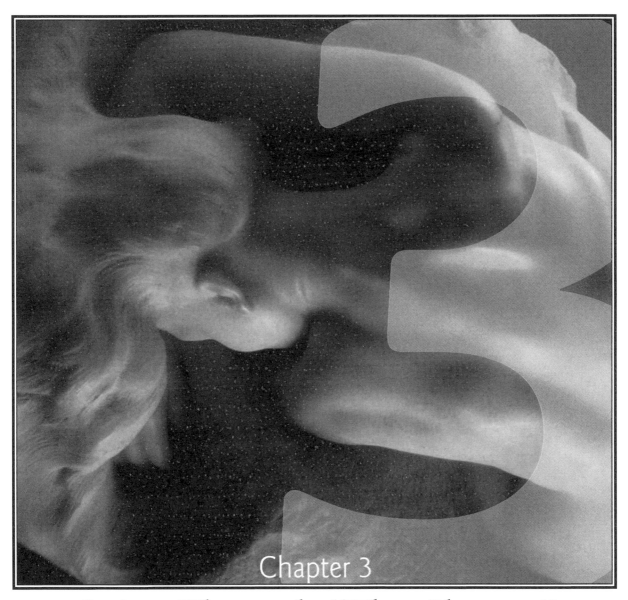

Chapter 3

Going Through "The Change"

Chapter 3
Going Through "The Change"

Mood swings, insomnia, irritability, a skipped period here and there. Are they signs that menopause is at hand, or simply the result of a too-hectic schedule, stress levels spun out of control, problems at work, or any of a host of other factors that can wreak havoc with the body's biological systems—in particular, hormone levels—and throw everything out of whack?

As is often the case when dealing with issues related to the chemistry of the body, there isn't one single answer to this question. However, when these symptoms appear in women of a certain age—over 40 years old—it's almost a sure bet that they are caused, at least in part, by the fluctuations in the sex hormones that signify the onset of menopause.

This period in a woman's life has been euphemistically referred to as "the change," "going through the change," or "the change of life" for about as long as anyone can remember. While these terms are a bit disin-genuous—as there really isn't a time when bodies aren't changing—they are pretty apt descriptions for what is more formally called perimenopause, which refers to the time leading up to when menstruation ceases.

During perimenopause, fundamental changes take place in how a woman's body secretes and processes the hormones needed for reproduction. These changes cause both emotional and physical symptoms—ranging from relatively benign to quite profound—that also change how a woman experiences life. The list of the changes that women's bodies go through is comprehensive and lengthy. None of the body's systems is unaffected.

If you don't realize that these changes—or symptoms—are part of perimenopause, a natural stage of life that virtually all women experience (the only exceptions being some women who go through surgical menopause), it can feel as if you're a stranger in your own body when you begin to experience them.

Since many of the symptoms are similar to those that characterize PMS, it can be easy to dismiss them. Not knowing that they are a part of perimenopause also leads many women into a frantic search for treatments and remedies that address individual symptoms instead of dealing with the underlying issue—the hormonal balance (or imbalance)—that is causing them.

Is it necessary to know exactly when "the change" starts? Not really. Being unable to pin down its exact onset isn't much of a cause for concern. Nor is it possible to predict exactly when it will begin, although a loose prediction can be based on the age that other women in your family experienced it. What we do know is that it can last for anywhere from five to 15 years before menstruation completely ceases, and its average duration is six years. During this time, the supply of follicles and eggs in the ovaries declines sharply and the pituitary gland tries to overcompensate for this decline by sending out increased amounts of hormones. This causes more severe hormonal fluctuations than usual, and these fluctuations are responsible for many of perimenopause's symptoms.

Knowing more about the symptoms of perimenopause, and what causes them, can help you recognize them for what they are and better prepare for them when they do arise. It can also help you know how to address and if necessary treat them. And, finally, it will help you know that what you are experiencing is very normal, even if it sometimes seems as if you've lost control of your body and your mind and you don't quite recognize yourself because of it.

Again, it's important to keep in mind that every woman experiences menopause in a different way. For some women, all hell breaks loose when their hormones start to shift. For others, the changes take place so gradually that they experience few if any symptoms at all. Also, no two women will experience symptoms in the same sequence. Some women realize that they're in perimenopause when they begin to have hot flashes or when their periods become irregular, which are two of the most classic indicators of the hormonal changes that take place during this time. Others will experience a host of other hormonally related issues, such as adult acne, increased facial hair, more frequent urinary-tract infections, or frequent urination, long before any of the more recognizable signs of perimenopause begin to manifest themselves.

I can't stress enough the importance of

taking a whole-body approach when addressing perimenopausal symptoms. The majority of the symptoms experienced during this period are either directly related to changes in hormone levels or affected by them, yet many medical professionals simply ignore the role that hormones play and treat the symptoms rather than the cause.

In saying this, I don't mean in any way to marginalize other medical conditions that call for treatment that goes beyond hormone therapy. Mood swings, depression, and anxiety, for example, can be related to hormonal imbalances that affect how the cells in the brain operate, or they can be caused by other chemical imbalances in the brain. A loss of interest in sex can be caused by certain medications, such as antidepressants, tranquilizers, and high-blood-pressure drugs. While addressing hormonal imbalances may improve these conditions, treatment often goes beyond this to include counseling, psychotherapy, and prescription-drug treatment.

When it comes to addressing the symptoms of perimenopause, a great deal of misdiagnosis goes on. If there are other factors present that can contribute to perimenopausal symptoms, it often seems sensible to attribute symptoms to those factors. If, on the other hand, there aren't, it's folly to go off on a wild goose chase in search of them and spend considerable amounts of time and money on a battery of diagnostic tests when a simple check of the hormones could tell a great deal.

Some medical professionals draw lines of distinction between symptoms that are most often correlated to menopause and those that can be caused by what they call the "natural aging process." I don't like this approach, because the distinction sets menopause apart from the aging process and therefore infers that it is a disease or illness and not part of the natural continuum of life. It is true that some of the changes women notice when they go through menopause—such as age spots on the skin, for example—are more directly related to aging (in this case, the photoaging that accumulates from years of sun exposure). Again, however, the majority of the symptoms experienced during this period are either directly related to changes in hormone levels or affected by them. Since they are, it's better not to attribute them to menopause or aging exclusively but instead to look at them as part of a normal stage in the aging process.

Perimenopausal Symptoms

As I have already mentioned, the list of various symptoms and associated conditions that women might experience during menopause is a long one. Below are some of the ones that are most frequently reported:

- acne
- allergies
- anxiety
- bloating
- blood sugar imbalances
- blurry vision
- bone loss
- breast tenderness
- depression
- dry eyes
- facial hair
- fatigue
- feelings of being imbalanced or out of control
- fibrocystic breasts
- food sensitivities
- fuzzy thinking

- hair thinning or loss
- headaches
- heart palpitations
- hot flashes
- hypothyroidism
- hysteria
- inability to lose weight
- insomnia
- irritability
- joint and back pain
- leg cramps
- loss of sexual desire
- menstrual cycle irregularities
- migraines
- memory problems
- mood swings
- muscle weakness
- night sweats
- panic attacks
- sagging breasts
- skin aging and dryness

▸ stomach upsets and cramps

▸ urinary frequency and/or urgency

▸ urinary incontinence

▸ urinary infections

▸ uterine fibroids

▸ vaginal dryness

▸ water retention

▸ weeping

▸ weight gain

▸ weight loss inability

Some of these symptoms—such as sagging breasts and dry skin—aren't health risks and are more along the lines of annoyances, things that women would rather not have to deal with but that can nonetheless be coped with if necessary. Others, such as bone loss, migraines, urinary-tract issues, and weight gain, present more serious medical issues that should be addressed as soon as possible to avoid more serious health problems in later years.

Of this long list of symptoms, some are more commonly experienced than others. Let's take a look at several of these in greater detail.

"I Just Don't Feel Like Myself"

For many women, one of the first signs of perimenopause is the realization that they simply don't feel the same or react to things in the same way as they used to. Women who were pretty much able to remain on an even keel in the past may find themselves feeling more irritable and less able to allow problems to roll off their backs. At times, emotions may whirl out of control over the slightest provocation. Attention spans often grow shorter. Some women describe a feeling of "fuzziness" in the

A recent study at Harvard Medical School found that women with a history of depression might enter perimenopause sooner than women who have never suffered from this mood disorder. Researchers analyzed data from 332 women with a history of major depression and 644 women without one. They found that women who suffered from chronic depression were 20 percent more likely to enter menopause early. Those who were most severely depressed were twice as likely to enter menopause sooner than their non-depressed peers.

Researchers theorized that depression affects the normal production of ovarian and brain hormones, which would bring about earlier than normal perimenopause. Stress was another contributing factor.

brain or say they feel as if they've suddenly developed attention deficit disorder. Experiencing mood swings, feeling "blue" or depressed, or feeling as though PMS systems are getting worse are other common complaints.

These symptoms are often linked to such other midlife stressors such as changes in family structure, career concerns, the health issues of a spouse, and fears over growing older. It can also be difficult to distinguish psychological changes related to menopause from more serious problems, such as depression.

According to the North American Menopause Society (NAMS), women with a history of psychiatric illness may have more problems with this illness during perimenopause. Women who experience depression during perimenopause are more likely to have had depressive episodes such as PMDD (premenstrual dysphoric disorder – the more serious form of premenstrual syndrome) or postpartum affective disorders.

Part of the cause for these symptoms has to do with how estrogen affects the brain. As discussed in Chapter 2, one of estrogen's functions is as a neurotransmitter regulator. Fluctuations in estrogen levels affect neuro-

transmitter uptake, which in turn affects how brain cells function and communicate with one other. At the same time, the brain needs to continue to receive messages from adequate levels of anabolic steroids—including DHEA, progesterone, androstenedione, testosterone, and dihydrotestosterone. The brain's myelin-producing schwann cells need these continuous messages from progesterone to optimize their nerve-protecting function. Selective serotonin reuptake inhibitors (SSRIs), which increase the availability of the neurotransmitter serotonin, are often prescribed for depression. These SSRI drugs work by keeping the serotonin released around the spaces called synapses of nerves cells longer than usual. The enzyme system designed to pull serotonin out of the synapse is blocked by medications like Paxil, Prozac, and Zoloft.

The SSRIs that contain fluorine are of particular concern to me. Flourine is one of the most powerful free-radical-oxidizing elements. In my opinion continued use of it simply cannot be safe. I suspect that these drugs may cause cortical atrophy and/or dementia problems after years of use. The FDA determines safety based only on short periods of drug testing before drugs are approved. The natural alternative to these drugs is tryptophan, which converts into more available serotonin without blocking or poisoning the naturally occurring enzymes designed to remove serotonin from the synapse. Balancing hormone levels—in the brain, estrogen has antidepressant qualities—can also help with these symptoms.

It is important to note that before menopause women may experience the severe premenstrual syndrome known as PMDD, mentioned above. PMDD's symptoms include severe monthly mood swings and physical symptoms that interfere with everyday life, especially a woman's relationships with her family and friends. PMDD symptoms go far beyond what are considered manageable or normal premenstrual symptoms.

PMDD is a combination of symptoms that may include irritability, depression, anxiety, sleep disturbance, difficulty in concentrating, angry outbursts, breast tenderness, and bloating. The condition affects up to one in 20 American women who have regular menstrual periods. Some women's symptoms can be so extreme that they feel suicidal during this second half of menstruation. Effective treatment is available and may include taking natural, bioavailable progesterone from around day 12 through day 25 of the menstrual cycle. Deficiencies in any or all of such essential

nutrients as amino acids, fatty acids, vitamins, and minerals (such as calcium, magnesium, selenium, chromium, lithium, and others) may be involved as well.

Irregular Menstrual Cycles/Changes in Bleeding

For many women, changes in their menstrual cycles are the first clues they have that they're going through menopause. They'll suddenly skip a cycle or two or experience any of various other changes, including the following:

- bleeding that is lighter or heavier than normal
- bleeding for fewer or more than four days
- cycles that are shorter or longer than normal

According to the NAMS, approximately 90 percent of women experience four to eight years of menstrual-cycle changes during perimenopause.

Vasomotor Symptoms

Commonly known as hot flashes and night sweats, these are among the most reported signs of perimenopause. According to the NAMS, they constitute the second-most-frequently-reported perimenopausal symptom, trailing only irregular periods, with as many as 85 percent of women having them. Interestingly, they are most common among Caucasians, with as many as 75 percent of Caucasian women reporting them.

The frequency and severity of hot flashes and night sweats differs widely between women. Some women get them hourly; others can go for months without having them. Most women who get them usually experience them for as long as three to five years, but some women report having them longer than this. For some, they can even continue well after menopause.

No one knows exactly what causes hot flashes, although it's believed that they're a result of the changes that take place in the hypothalamus (the part of the brain that regulates body temperature). Something causes the hypothalamus to mis-

takenly conclude that the body is too warm. When it does, it causes a series of physical reactions that are designed to cool things down. It's also known that estrogen receptors exist in the smooth-muscle walls of the arteries. When estrogen levels drop, the smooth muscles relax, causing dilation of the arteries, and thus hot-flash symptoms may occur. Therefore, hot flashes are considered by most to be an estrogen-deficiency symptom. Some women report a reduction in hot flashes after taking progesterone alone. Some researchers have reported that small amounts of progesterone may be converted to estrogen in the body.

Factors known to commonly trigger hot flashes include the following:

▶ experiencing stress

▶ being in a warm room

▶ using a hair dryer or other styling aids, such as hot rollers and flat irons, that heat up the scalp

▶ eating hot or

HOT

A hot flash will make you feel, well, hot, but in fact your core body temperature actually drops when you have them. This happens due to the heat lost through evaporative cooling (perspiration) and increased blood flow to the skin, resulting in your feeling chilled. Some women experience chills without an accompanying hot flash.

Hot-flash Help

● Stick to natural fabrics in clothing and bedding.

● Sleep in a cool room.

● Wear layers of clothes and remove some when you get warm.

● When a hot flash starts, grab a cool drink.

● Avoid alcohol.

spicy foods

▸ imbibing in hot drinks

▸ using caffeine

▸ drinking alcohol

▸ taking certain medications

For most women, hot flashes and night sweats affect their quality of life to some extent. Some hot flashes are relatively transient and easy to ignore, but they can also leave a woman flushed and drenched in sweat—which disrupts both daily activities and sleep quality.

Hot flashes are the leading reason for women to seek professional help during perimenopause. Estrogen therapy is often prescribed. While fluctuating hormone levels are almost always the culprit, there are other, albeit rare, causes for them, including thyroid disorders, infections, leukemia, mast-cell disorders, autoimmune disorders, and pancreatic tumors.

Sleep Disorders

Sleeplessness and fitful sleep are common during perimenopause. Ranging from transient—lasting for just a few days or so—to

Sleep Suggestions

Many women find that creating a regular evening routine that might include going to bed at the same time every night and drinking something warm, like a noncaffeinated herbal tea or warm milk, helps them to get back to a normal sleep cycle. Be sure to keep the bedroom at a comfortable temperature and avoid alcohol, large meals, caffeine, and working too close to bedtime, all of which many women find interferes with getting a good night's sleep. You may find that sticking to a regular 30 minutes of physical exercise on most days of the week will help you sleep. Be sure to avoid napping during the day.

chronic, these symptoms can have a significant effect on one's quality of life. Diminished quality of sleep—that is, not sleeping well, and not getting enough sleep—has been linked to a number of problems, including the following:

▸ lethargy

▸ inability to concentrate

▸ tension and irritability

▸ chronic illnesses, such as cardiac problems and depression, tension and irritability

Night sweats contribute to sleep problems during perimenopause, but they're not the

A Vaginal-dryness Tip

You can help to relieve vaginal dryness and irritation by using an over-the-counter vaginal lubricant. Some women find that Vitamin E works well for them. If you use condoms make sure that whatever lubricant you choose is latex friendly.

only cause. Stress and chronic illnesses can also bring about spates of sleepless nights.

According to the National Sleep Foundation, perimenopausal and post-menopausal women sleep less, experience insomnia more frequently, and are more than twice as likely to use prescription sleeping aids. But these figures are probably extremely low. Most people—both men and women—don't talk to their doctors about sleep problems, and most doctors don't ask about them either.

My Aching Head

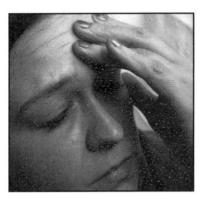

Headaches, ranging from mild to severe, are often more common during perimenopause. While there are many causes for them, such as sinus problems, stress, eyestrain, dehydration, allergies, and food sensitivities, some research points to hormonal fluctuations as

causing headaches that occur more frequently and are more severe. Women who experience headaches related to their menstrual cycles often find that their headaches become more frequent, more severe, or both during menopause.

"Not Tonight, Dear"

The hormonal fluctuations of perimenopause cause physical and psychological changes that often affect sexual desire and function. How much they change varies greatly depending on the individual, but many women report problems in this area, including a lower sex drive, less responsiveness, and physical discomfort during sex.

Sexual matters are always complex, and there are a number of factors that can contribute to problems here. However, some experts believe that lower estrogen levels, which can cause changes in the cardiovascular system (affecting arterial blood flow) and the central and peripheral nervous systems (affecting touch and vibration perception), can be responsible for at least part of the problem.

Declining estrogen levels also cause rapid changes in the lining of the vagina, as well as slower changes to the vagina's vascular, muscular, and connective tissues. These changes affect normal arousal responses and cause the vagina to lose elasticity, which can result in painful intercourse.

When it comes to the desire to have sex, declining androgens, and specifically testosterone, get the blame. Testosterone drives motivation, desire, and sexual sensation in both men and women. Although men produce far greater quantities of it than women do, when it declines desire goes along with it for both sexes.

In women, androgen insufficiency is believed to be responsible for between 30 percent and 50 percent of sexual-dysfunction issues.

Symptoms of declining testosterone levels include the following:

▸ lower energy levels in general

▸ less sexual desire

▸ diminishment in one's ability to achieve orgasm

▸ decreased nipple and clitoral sensitivity

▸ decreased muscle tone

▸ dry skin

▸ thinning of pubic hair

During menopause, decreases in sex-hormone-binding globulin (SHBG) take place in some women. When they do, however, testosterone levels actually increase, as SHBG binds with both estrogen and testosterone. However, oral estrogens increase SHBG levels—with the end result being lower free testosterone and lower sexual desire.

Lower progesterone levels don't appear to affect sexual functioning, although women have reported occasional increases in libido from natural-progesterone therapy. However, some types of progesterone therapy can affect mood negatively or cause uterine bleeding; both of these developments can contribute to changes in sexual function and/or activity.

By the time most women reach their middle 40s, their testosterone levels have already decreased by anywhere from 10 percent to 50 percent. During menopause, testosterone production continues to decrease again by one-third to one-half.

Vaginal Changes

Estrogen loss often causes decreases in vaginal fluid. It also changes one's pH balance from acidic to alkaline, which can increase susceptibility for vaginal irritation and infection.

A more serious estrogen-related problem is vaginal atrophy. It begins with thinning of the vaginal walls and eventually causes decreases in elasticity, vaginal blood flow, and cervical and vaginal secretions, all of which will result in decreased lubrication. The vagina also narrows and shortens. In some women, vaginal walls develop chronic inflammation and petechiae—small, round red or purple spots caused by hemorrhages in the skin or mucous membranes.

All of these changes increase the chances of injury and infection and of pain during intercourse. Keeping sexually active reduces the chances of one's experiencing them.

Urinary-tract Problems

The urethra and the bladder also contain estrogen receptors. Therefore, they too are affected by falling estrogen levels during peri-menopause. As levels diminish, a portion of the urethra shortens and shrinks—minimizing its ability to defend against pathogens and increasing the risk of urinary-tract infections.

Test Early and Test Often

I recommend that all of my female patients have their hormone levels tested as soon as possible when they feel they've reached perimenopause. Doing so provides a baseline that later tests can be compared to, and better monitoring of hormone levels over time.

Urinary incontinence also becomes more common during perimenopause, due to thinning of the bladder walls and reduced smooth-muscle tone.

Thinning of the uterine and the bladder walls also takes place during perimenopause, and both organs become somewhat smaller. This effect is more pronounced as estrogen levels continue to drop throughout the post-menopausal years in women without estrogen replacement or adequate gland-estrogen reserves and utilization.

Some women report the need to urinate more frequently; others have sudden urges to urinate even though the bladder may not be full. Other problems include urinating during the night when asleep; leaking urine when coughing, sneezing, laughing, or lifting or during sexual intercourse or orgasm; and painful urination.

How to Know if You're Really Going Through the Change

If you're experiencing the more obvious signs of perimenopause, such as hot flashes, night sweats, irregular periods, and so on, there's probably not much question in your mind as to whether or not you're going through the change. If your symptoms are subtler, you might be tempted to chalk them up to the other factors discussed at the beginning of this chapter. But if you want to know for sure, you can have your hormone levels tested.

The most common diagnostic tests for perimenopause measure the blood levels of follicle-stimulating hormone (FSH) and luteinizing hormone (LH) respectively. These tests work well as an indication of menopause itself, as the levels of both are elevated during it. However, they are inadequate on their own for diagnosing perimenopause, as they can both fluctuate greatly during this period, which can result in misdiagnosis.

In order to get the most accurate picture of what's going on, it's important to also test for the levels of the sex hormones—the three estrogens (estrone, estradiol, and estriol), plus progesterone and testosterone. These levels also fluctuate quite a bit, so it's necessary to have each test repeated more than once. Some physicians advise having all the tests done at the same time and on the same day of your menstrual cycle. Others recommend doing them on different days to get a better idea of how much levels fluctuate. As baseline testing, I'll usually screen thyroid function with a

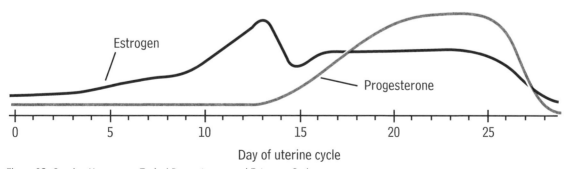

Figure 13: Ovarian Hormones - Typical Progesterone and Estrogen Cycle

TSH, measure the other steroids and androgens with a 24-hour-urinary hormone test, and measure IGF1 as a marker for a possible growth-hormone deficiency. If the 24-hour urinary-hormone test indicates you have a low level of DHEA, you are more likely to be low in IGF1 and growth hormone as well.

For more information on testing and monitoring, turn to Chapter 12.

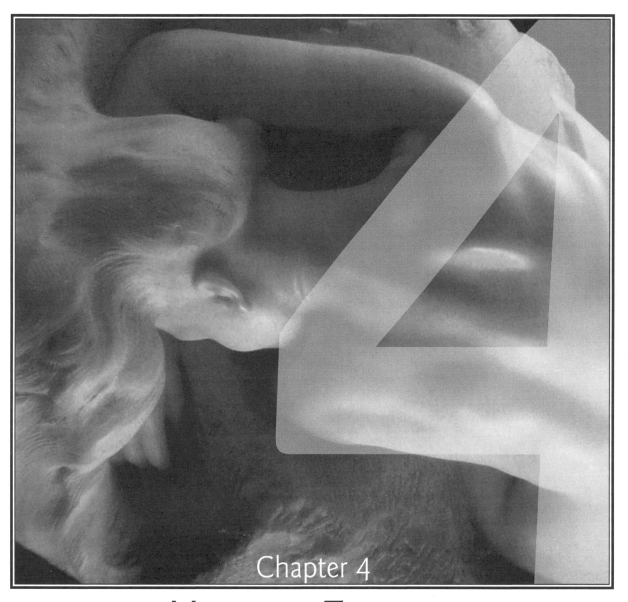

Chapter 4

Menopause Treatment:
Conventional Medicine's Approach

Chapter 4

Menopause Treatment: Conventional Medicine's Approach

When women decide to do something to help manage their own passage through perimenopause and to head off health problems that can occur after menopause, more often than not they end up seeking the advice of their primary-care physicians. For more than three decades, the solution preferred by modern medicine revolved around one main approach: boosting declining hormone levels with synthetic or non-molecularly bioidentical hormones. Doing so relieved such discomforts as hot flashes, vaginal dryness, and mood swings during perimenopause. After menopause, it appeared to protect women from cardiovascular disease and osteoporosis, which are, of course, two of the leading causes of death in older women.

This wasn't a bad approach on the face of it, and it was believed that any downside or risks associated with it were outweighed by its lifesaving benefits. Over time, however, research has proven this approach to be badly flawed. While there's little doubt that it offers some benefits, many experts now believe that it may have done more damage than good.

Balancing the Body

When something is lacking, it only makes sense to replace it. This is the theory behind using hormones to manage the symptoms of menopause.

Of the hormones in a woman's body, estrogen was initially identified as the most important to replace. For this reason, early treatment focused on this hormone alone. Premarin, the first estrogen pill, was introduced in 1942. Following its release, several studies were done that supported the use of supplemental estrogen. One determined that hormone replacement might enhance verbal memory in elderly women. In 1959, the *Journal of the American Medical Association* reported on the results of a 25-year study that reinforced the benefits of prolonged estrogen therapy.

The researchers found that estrogen protected bones and relieved the troubling symptoms of menopause. They further found that any concerns over breast and cervical cancer related to estrogen therapy appeared to be unfounded.

> According to the Humane Society of the United States there are approximately 500 Premarin farms in North America. As millions of women from the "baby boom" generation enter menopause this number is expected to rise.

Estrogen therapy didn't garner a great deal of attention until the mid-60s. At that time, a gynecologist named Robert Wilson popularized the idea that estrogen could rejuvenate women who had reached "a certain age" (read "menopause").

Wilson, who had previously reported in a *JAMA* article that taking estrogen during menopause reduced breast and genital cancers, wrote a best-selling book called <u>Feminine Forever</u>, which was published in 1966. In it, he described women who were going through menopause as "vapid cows," occupying crumbling, decaying bodies caused by decreasing estrogen levels.

Since women were clearly of little value to their families or their husbands in such states, Wilson suggested that their only hope of regaining any semblance of their earlier functionality and beauty was to take supplemental estrogen, which would magically transform them into younger-looking, more attractive women who felt better, looked better, and were better able to meet the needs of their families.

"From a purely biologic point of view," Wilson wrote, "estrogen therapy can hardly be regarded as altering the natural state of life. On the contrary, as we have pointed out before, it merely restores a natural harmony

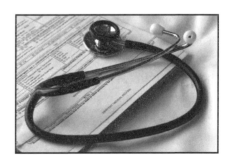

between the rate of aging and life expectancy, a harmony that has been disturbed by the lengthened lifespan of modern women. It is the case of the untreated woman—the prematurely aging castrate—that is unnatural."

Although Premarin's manufacturer disputes this, a number of sources state that Wilson had strong ties to the pharmaceutical company and that they may have underwritten both his research and the book. What isn't disputable is that the manufacturer mounted a massive marketing campaign that coincidentally accompanied the book's release, aimed at convincing women that taking supplemental estrogen would keep them from turning into menopausal "castrates." Not only that, but they were promised relief from menopause's discomforts, including hot flashes and vaginal pain, as well as protection from cardiovascular disease and osteoporosis.

Millions of women (and their physicians) rushed to embrace what appeared to be a miracle cure for the ravages of aging. As they did, they gave little thought to the possibility that there might be some downsides to the treatment. By 1970, almost 14 million prescriptions for Premarin were dispensed. Most women who went on estrogen replacement therapy reported that they felt better with hormone therapy than without it. Their symptoms went away, and they felt more like themselves again. Taking hormones also put their minds at ease about having to cope with heart disease and osteoporosis in the future. Some women reported minor irritations, things like fluid retention, bloating, headache, nausea, anxiety, and irritability, but these were considered bearable compared to what life would be like without estrogen. They were minor concerns when weighed against estrogen's lifesaving benefits.

In an interview in 2003 Ronald Wilson, son of gynecologist and author of Feminine Forever Robert Wilson, stated that the pharmaceutical giant that manucatures Premarin paid his father for the writing of the book, covered the cost of opening an office on Park Avenue for the doctor, and sponsored speeches that he made. A spokesman for the drug manufacturer says there is no evidence of a financial relationship between Ronald Wilson and themselves.

The Downside Surfaces

In the mid-70s, the first indications that estrogen therapy might not be a magic cure began to appear. A clinical trial of men taking Premarin to prevent heart attacks and strokes was stopped when the frequency of heart attacks and blood clots increased in the study group. In 1975, two studies published in the *New England Journal of Medicine* reported that using estrogen after menopause increased the risk for endometrial cancer four to 14 times. By 1979, the journal was reporting on a study that found that women who had never used estrogen had less than one-tenth the risk of developing endometrial cancer that users had. In 1976, the *New England Journal of Medicine* published the first study that showed a link between menopausal estrogen and breast cancer. However, the medical community continued to believe that the benefits of the therapy outweighed the risks.

Enter Progesterone

In 1980, an article in *Obstetrics and Gynecology* reported that combining progestin (synthetic progesterone), which could block or oppose estrogen's cancer-causing tenden-

cies, with estrogen led to a decline in endometrial cancer. Finally, physicians began prescribing both of the hormones that were involved in regulating a woman's menstrual cycle.

The progesterone prescribed by most physicians was Provera, another synthetic non-biologically-identical hormone. However, Provera was only successful in minimizing the risk of endometrial cancer. It did nothing to mitigate breast cancer. In 1989, a Swedish study of more than 23,000 women, the results of which were published in the *New England Journal of Medicine*, showed a slight increase in breast cancer among the women who used only estrogen. For the women who took the combination therapy, breast-cancer risk more than doubled.

Still more studies confirmed earlier reports that estrogen might do more harm than good. But conflicting data began to surface. The Nurse's Health Study, based on questionnaires sent to more than 100,000 female nurses age 30 to 55, concluded that the risk of coronary heart disease stopped in those who took estrogen. Of the more than 32,000 study participants, coronary-disease rates were roughly half those of nurses who had never taken estrogen.

A Framingham Heart Study report published the same year stated that cardiovascular problems in women taking estrogen were 50 percent higher than in those who didn't. The results of a Swedish study released in 1989 also raised concerns about breast-cancer increases among women who were on combined HRT. The study also noted that cancer rates appeared to be higher due to progestins, the first time that this correlation was made.

Still, hormone replacement therapy that used synthetic hormones continued to be the premier approach to managing menopausal symptoms. By the 1990s, Premarin was the most frequently dispensed prescription drug in the United States. Wyeth, Premarin's manufacturer, also petitioned the FDA for changing Premarin's label so the company could include wording advising that Premarin could be used to prevent heart disease in women without a uterus. Although an advisory committee voted for the change, the FDA didn't approve it—based on a lack of hard data supporting Premarin's cardiovascular benefits.

Then, in 1991, hormone replacement ther-apy was again put to the test with the launching of the Women's Health Initiative (WHI), a long-term, national study of women and their health sponsored by the National Institutes of Health (NIH) and the National Heart, Lung, and Blood Institute (NHLBI). Involving more than 161,000 women ages 50 to 79, it was heralded as one of the most definitive, far-reaching clinical trials of women's health ever undertaken in the United States.

Since the study was designed to address many of the inequities in women's-health research, results would be used to provide solid, practical information to women and their physicians in three areas: hormone replacement therapy, dietary patterns, and calcium and vitamin D supplementation.

The first component examined the effect of HRT (in this case, Premarin and synthetic progesterone) on the prevention of heart disease and osteoporosis, as well as any associated risk for breast cancer.

> It's important to note that the WHI study and almost all the other studies not only used Premarin and synthetic progesterone, but used them in doses that were not monitored and were not adjusted to pre- and post-hormone lab levels.

"We Were Wrong"

In 1995, Wyeth introduced Prempro, the first estrogen/progestin combo pill, making it easier for women to be compliant when combined hormone therapy was prescribed. To support its new product, the company funded a four-year heart-disease-prevention trial called the Heart and Estrogen/Progestin Replacement Study (HERS).

About a year into the study, investigators met to review the data they had collected to date. In so doing, they found substantial differences between the two groups of women being studied, with one group experiencing far greater incidences of cardiovascular problems, including heart attacks, blood clots, and pulmonary embolisms, than the other. When the data was unmasked, investigators found that the problems related not to the placebo group, as they had thought, but to the women who were on HRT.

Although the study's investigators considered canceling the trial, it was allowed to continue. Findings reported in 1998 showed that HRT had not been effective in reducing coronary heart disease in women. What's more, HRT had actually increased the rate of blood

clots and gallbladder disease. In fact, there had been a 50 percent increase in cardiovascular events in the first year of HERS. This had leveled off, but the final verdict was clear: HRT didn't protect these women from heart disease. In fact, it did quite the opposite.

Similar findings were beginning to surface in the WHI study, which was testing two types of hormone therapy: estrogen only for women who had had hysterectomies and combination estrogen/progestin therapy for those who hadn't. At about the same time that the HERS results were announced, WHI officials were advising study participants of increased incidents of heart attacks, strokes, and blood clots among HRT users.

By 2002, an estimated 6 million American women were using estrogen and progestin to treat hot flashes and other menopausal symptoms and to prevent bone loss. Many also believed, based on what their physicians told them and on what they had read, that such treatment also protected them from cardiovascular disease and heart attacks. By this time, the WHI study was also turning up disturbing findings linking breast cancer to HRT—with a 26 percent increased risk of cancer among women taking the combination therapy. Coupled with the previous data that reflected even higher risks of strokes and heart attacks, the Prempro arm of the study was halted in July 2002.

Although the adverse effects of HRT had been reported previously, the halting of the WHI study caused a maelstrom. The news that HRT, which so many women had relied on to keep them healthy, could indeed put them at greater risk for developing serious health problems, called into question the entire theory of hormone replacement therapy. In its aftermath, countless numbers of women stopped undergoing combined-hormone treatment. Some stopped all forms of hormone therapy and decided to pursue other courses of action, ranging from doing nothing to exploring alternative treatments.

As mentioned, the findings in the WHI study confirmed those reached in the majority of other investigations; the only notable exception was the Nurses' Health Study. Researchers still don't know why the two studies reached such disparate conclusions, but the answer may simply reflect the differences between the parameters for each study and the populations that participated in them.

As analyses of the WHI study's findings have continued, it is becoming increasingly clear that there is no one best course of action when it comes to treating menopausal symptoms. Many practitioners of conventional medicine believe that HRT's benefits, including reduced risks of hip fractures and colorectal cancer, continue to outweigh the risks of combination therapy, as the increased risk shown by the study is actually quite small. Others believe that HRT continues to be an important tool in preventing coronary heart disease, though not for women who exhibit certain risk factors, such as elevated cholesterol and blood pressure, that would make them susceptible to heart problems if they were to take oral estrogen.

In October 2002, the North American Menopause Society (NAMS) issued a set of recommendations that reflected the medical community's uncertainty regarding HRT. In short, the recommendations suggested that a risk-benefit analysis was "essential for every postmenopausal woman contemplating any regimen of hormone replacement therapy" and that hormone supplements should be limited to treating symptoms like hot flashes and vaginal dryness.

It was also recommended that for those

women who still want hormone therapy, physicians should prescribe lower-than-standard doses for the shortest period of time, that hormones should not be used to help prevent heart disease, and that alternative medications should be considered to prevent osteoporosis. Finally, the NAMS announced that it was appointing a panel of experts that will take a critical look at the existing research and try to sort out the confusion that resulted from it.

Close on the heels of the NAMS recommendations came a separate set from the U.S. Preventive Services Task Force, which in November 2002 recommended against the routine use of combination therapy for preventing chronic conditions in postmenopausal women, based on "fair to good evidence" that the increased risk for breast cancer, strokes, blood clots, and gallbladder problems outweigh the chronic-disease-prevention benefits in most women. As the NAMS did before it, the task force also stressed that the decision to use conventional hormone therapy should be an individual choice and that individual risk factors and the presence of menopausal symptoms should have strong bearing on whether such therapy was prescribed.

Such recommendations underscore a truth that the conventional medical community has ignored for a long time: When it comes to treating the individual, a "one size fits all" approach simply doesn't work. While the reasons for allowing this philosophy to continue for as long as it has when it comes to treating women for menopausal symptoms can be debated, it's clear that we have now moved into a new era when it comes to how a woman's menopausal symptoms are viewed and managed.

> A study, the results of which appeared in the December 2002 issue of *Obstetrics and Gynecology* reported some good news for women, as it found that the risk of breast cancer diminishes six months after women stop HRT. Still, it also recommended against long-term combination hormonal therapy and stated that any therapy should be limited to treating hot flashes for the shortest amount of time and in the lowest possible dosages.

With this new era has also come a new name for hormone therapy, thanks to the NIH, which in late October 2002 announced that HRT would thereafter be called "menopausal hormone therapy", as a reflection of the fact that it was never meant to be a "replacement" and shouldn't be presented as a way to restore a woman's youth.

While this new moniker has yet to catch on, it does symbolize an important shift in focus that many would argue is long overdue. Rather than viewing menopause as a time in a woman's life when it's necessary to boost hormone levels to what they were when she was young, it's instead being thought of more as it should be: as a natural stage of a woman's aging process. Now, thanks to this, instead of hormone replacement therapy's being viewed

as the key approach to managing menopausal symptoms, it is being positioned more as one of many approaches a woman can choose.

With this said, the array of manufactured synthetic estrogens and progestins available to the prescribing physician, and his patient, is daunting. The table below lists these estrogens and progestins/progesterones.

Current Manufactured Prescription Menopausal Hormone Therapy

Current Oral Combinations
- Premphase
- Prempro
- Fem HRT
- Ortho-Prefest
- Activella

Oral Estrogens
- Cenestin
- Estratab
- Premarin (conjugated equine estrogens)
- Estrace
- Ortha-Est
- Menest
- Ogen
- Gynediol

Progestins
- Provera
- Micronor
- Cycrin
- Amen
- Aygestin

Transdermal Estrogens
- Estraderm
- Vivelle
- Alora
- Estradiol
- Climara
- FemPatch
- Esclim

Progesterone
- Prometrium
- Crinone

Combination Transdermal
- CombiPatch
- Estradiol
- Vaginal Estrogen Creams
- Estrace cream
- Premarin cream
- Ogen cream
- Vagifem
- Estring

Table 4: Current Manufactured Prescription Menopausal Hormone Therapy

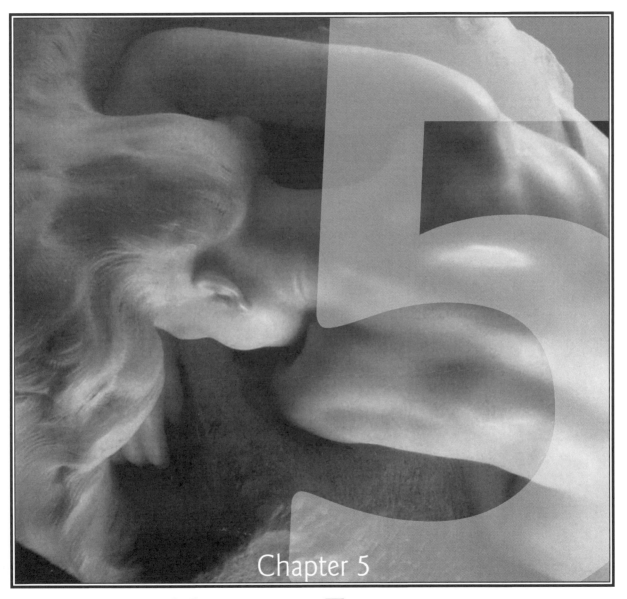

Chapter 5

Menopause Treatment:
The Natural-hormone-therapy Approach

Chapter 5

Menopause Treatment: The Natural-hormone-therapy Approach

When concerns over the long-term health risks of hormone replacement therapy came to a head when the Women's Health Initiative study was halted in 2002, many women who were taking the drugs, and those considering replacement therapy, were left in the lurch, not knowing what they should do next. Later the estrogen-only arm of the study was halted when investigators determined that women using this therapy were at an increased risk of strokes with no clear benefits in terms of prevention of heart disease, leaving women even more confused.

What many of them didn't realize—and quite possibly still don't—is that they do have an alternative to conventional hormones if they want to continue hormone therapy. Natural hormones—that is, hormones that are chemical replicas of the ones made by the human body—will deliver the same benefits—in fact, many believe better benefits—without the side effects associated with conjugated estrogens derived from horse urine.

Although natural hormone therapy has garnered more attention in the months following the release of the WHI findings, it still isn't a headline grabber. Part of the reason for this is that this therapy isn't exactly part of mainstream medicine. While natural hormones have been available for more than 20 years, many conventional physicians are unfamiliar with them and do not prescribe them. This wasn't a bad approach on the face of it, and it was believed that any downside or risks associated with it were outweighed by its lifesaving benefits. Over time, however, research has proven this approach to be badly flawed. While there's little doubt that it offers some benefits, many experts now believe that it may have done more damage than good.

When it comes to hormone therapy, it's far easier to put women on standardized doses of brand-name premanufactured products than it is to use natural hormones to custom-tailor a treatment regimen that addresses each women's specific needs, which, of course, is what natural hormone replacement is all about.

The other reason why natural hormone therapy is often overlooked is that there are no big drug companies promoting this approach. Because natural hormones are derived from a commonly available substance—wild yam—and are made to be the bioequivalent to human hormones, they aren't patentable. Equilin the horse estrogen that is used to make conjugated estrogens, is altered in the laboratory just enough to make it different from naturally occurring estrogen; consequently, it can be—and is—patented.

Detractors also point to the fact that there are few studies that specifically explore how natural hormones work in the body. This is certainly true in the United States, where most of the hormone studies are financed by grants from the makers of the hormone products

derived synthetically or from conjugated horse hormone. However, it's a different case in other countries, where studies have shown natural hormones to be as effective, if not better, than synthetic forms.

Bioidentical hormone replacement therapy offers a proven approach to both managing menopausal symptoms and promoting long-term health that may very well be the answer for women who want to continue taking hormones but are concerned over the health risks associated with conventional HRT, as well as for those women who simply feel safer using a natural alternative. It's the approach I and other doctors with similar philosophies have taken over the years with our patients who desire and need this treatment.

It's also an approach that I believe will become more popular—and that growing numbers of women will demand—as concerns over the negative effects of horse estrogens on the body continue to surface. As you will read later, this natural-hormone therapy becomes even safer when utilized in tandem with optimal laboratory testing.

What Are "Natural"* Hormones?

Natural, or bioidentical, hormones are hormones that are carbon copies of the hormones that the body normally produces, such as estrone, estradiol, estriol, progesterone, and testosterone.

While it is possible to synthesize these hormones from human urine, since they are excreted in it, wild yam, which is a vastly more accessible and plentiful substance, contains the molecule diosgenin—a naturally occurring precursor to estrogen—from which other molecules identical to the ones found in the human body can be formed. However, diosgenin can't be directly converted into bioidentical estrogens or progesterone in the body. It can only be done in a laboratory.

While diosgenin is still used to manufacture estrogen for humans, pregnant mares' urine has proven to be a cheaper and more abundant source. However, the estrogens in conjugated estrogen drugs that are made from horse urine also contain equilins. These estrogens are biochemically different from, and in some cases much stronger than, human estrogens. The human body doesn't contain all the enzymes

Bioidentical or Natural Hormones

- Estradiol
- Estrone
- Estriol
- Progesterone
- Testosterone

* You will often see hormones derived from wild yam, as well as from other plant sources of estrogen, such as soy, referred to as "natural hormones." However, so are the hormones derived from horse urine sometimes described as natural, because they are synthesized from a naturally occurring substance, not created from chemicals in a lab. For this reason, the two different types of hormones are often confused or lumped together as being natural.

The confusion over what is and isn't a "natural" hormone boils down to the liberal use of the word "natural" in alternative menopause therapies. When describing replacement hormones, practitioners prefer to reserve the word "natural" to describe the structure of the hormone, not its source. Here, I'll follow the intended use of the word "natural"—to describe the bioidentical hormones derived from wild yam.

Wild yam is by no means a new-comer to the world of herbal remedies. Native Americans have long used the root of this tuberous vine to treat colic (hence wild yam's other common name, colic root) as well as inflammation, muscle spasms, and asthma. Herbalists in the 18th and 19th centuries used it to treat menstrual cramps and problems related to childbirth.

The discovery in the 1940s that wild yam contains diosgenin, a steroid-like substance that can be used in the chemical synthesis of progesterone and estrogen, made possible the development of commercially available hormones and the birth-control pill. However, it's the chemical diosgenin that the plant contains that holds all the power. Since humans can't convert diosgenin into progesterone, eating the plant itself will have no beneficial effect. The same goes for "natural" progesterone creams that are made from wild yam. Only if they contain progesterone will they have any benefit. Over-the-counter progesterone creams can contain up to 2% (20 mg per gram) of natural progesterone without having to be "prescribed."

needed to completely metabolize these hormones. As a result, they remain in the body longer and produce estrogenic results that can lead to serious problems.

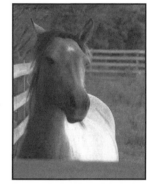

What's more, I, along with countless others, believe that manufacturing estrogen drugs from pregnant mares' urine is a highly unethical practice, because of the abuse that these mares are put through. They are, in effect, turned into "urine factories," kept constantly pregnant and confined to narrow stalls with galvanized buckets placed beneath them to collect as much urine as possible. They have zero quality of life. The idea is already troubling, but it becomes even more so when you consider that there are viable alternatives that are all but being ignored.

Plants that contain diosgenin are a far better choice, in terms of both bioequivalence and bioethics. Demand for the Dioscorea species, which wild yam belongs to, has caused excessive harvesting of some of these plants, but it has also led to the cultivation of other diosgenin-containing plants.

The Benefits of Using Natural Hormones

Proponents of hormones derived from pregnant mares' urine have argued (and continue to do so) that a hormone that is pretty close to that naturally found in the human body can be "good enough." Research, however, has shot down this claim. As discussed in greater detail in Chapter 2, these substances are indeed close to the real thing but simply don't work in the same way. Here's why: Hormones, the chemical messengers that the body produces to regulate certain processes, are all fashioned differently so that they will only link up with the cells that they're supposed to affect.

For example, thyroid-stimulating hormone, or TSH, will only bind to receptors on the surface of thyroid cells. Growth hormone, or GH, only binds to receptors on the surface of liver cells.

As detailed in Chapter 2, hormones like estrogen, progesterone, and testosterone are members of the steroid group, a large hormone group that has numerous effects on the body. Their chemical composition allows them to enter freely into all cells and the cell nucleus effecting DNA communication. However, like the other hormones, they only work the way they're supposed to when they enter target cells and nuclear DNA with receptors that are designed to bind with them.

It is possible to shape synthetic-drug molecules to mimic the action of natural hormones, but the key word here is "mimic." While they can be a near perfect fit, they can only come close. For this reason, synthetic hormones won't interact with the cells of the body in exactly the same way. They might overstimulate a cell's intended action or ask the cell to do more things than it should. Some can even alter the composition of receptor sites, causing them to resist binding to hormones that arc a perfect fit.

These molecules are also just different enough that the enzymes produced by the receptor cells that would normally help process them work improperly if at all. Instead of synthesizing into substances that the body can properly dispose of, they turn into substances that the body can only partially get rid of.

Natural hormones, on the other hand, work in the body as they're supposed to. They

Research from the Postmenopausal Estrogen/Progesterone Interventions (PEPI) study, the results of which appear in the November 2002 issue of the *Journal of Obstetrics and Gynecology*, found that women taking natural progesterone had far less bleeding than women taking a synthetic version of the same hormone. The study compared micronized progesterone (MP), which is chemically identical to naturally produced progesterone, to medroxyprogesterone acetate, or MPA, which was the synthetic progesterone used in the Women's Health Institute study.

are metabolized as they should be (if the person has a healthy liver), which means that they won't upset the balance of other hormones or produce a greater or lesser effect than they should. Natural hormones, when given in appropriate doses, relieve symptoms better than synthetic hormones do. They'll also protect against such long-term health concerns as osteoporosis and heart disease better than synthetic hormones can.

What's more, unlike synthetic hormones, natural estrogens and progesterone are compounded based on each patient's individual needs, leading to fewer side effects.

Are natural hormones right for you? This is a decision that you alone can make. But before dismissing all forms of hormone replacement therapy, it's worth checking out. Are there downsides to this form of therapy? Yes, but they're fairly minimal when compared with the risks involved with synthetic hormones. It can be more difficult to find a health-care professional who will prescribe them and, just as important, monitor your progress while, you're taking them. See the resources section at the end of this book for further support.

Depending on your medical coverage, they can be more expensive as well. Some insurance companies will cover the costs, but others might cover only part or even none. Natural hormone treatment can cost from $30 to $60 per month, but in my experience even women who have to cover all costs themselves generally feel that the expense is worth it.

Using Natural Hormones

Natural-hormone therapy involves taking the three forms of estrogen, progesterone, and testosterone (although not all women need testosterone, which I'll expand on shortly) that occur naturally in the body. Some women may also require additional hormonal augmentation to feel their best. This might include taking thyroid medication, DHEA, low-dose cortisol, and/or products called secretagogues to stimulate the release of growth hormone from the pituitary.

Why is it important to take all of these hormones? Because varying levels of all of them are naturally found in the body. Furthermore, when it comes to estrogens, there are subtle differences in their chemical compositions that cause them to have slightly different effects in the body, and to be metabolized differently.

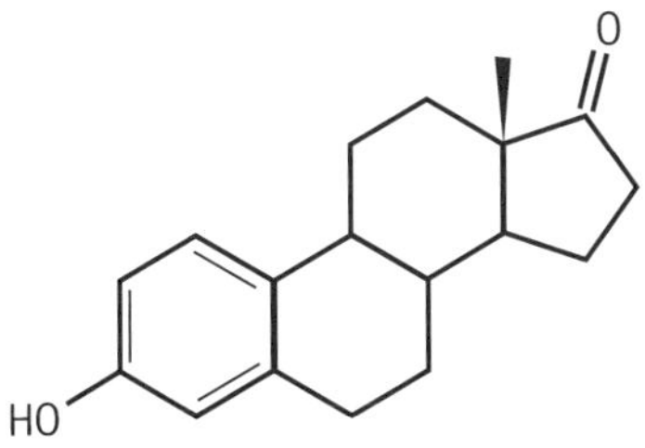

Estrone, or E1, is the dominant estrogen after menopause and is produced by fat cells after ovarian function declines. It has the same effects on the body that estradiol does but is weaker. Estradiol, or E2, is the most potent estrogen, and the one that is produced in the largest amounts during a woman's childbearing years, which means that levels of this hormone fall after menopause. It is extremely effective for relieving hot flashes and urinary-tract problems and for general well-being. The brain has a higher proportion of estradiol receptors, and estradiol seems to be the most effective in menopausal cognitive impairment.

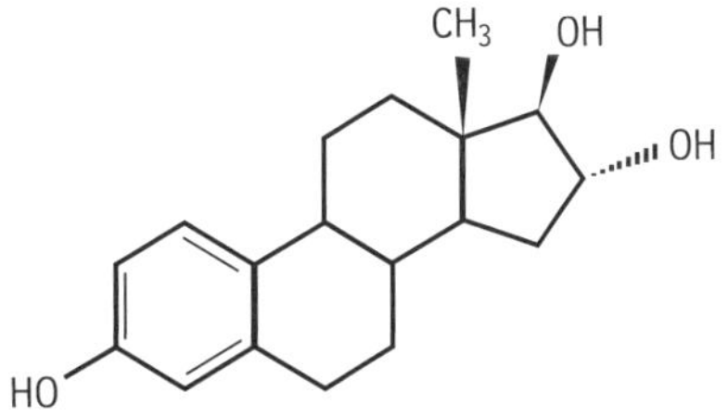

Figure 15: Estriol

Estriol, or E3, is the weakest of the three major estrogens. It is made in large quantities by the placenta during pregnancy and is also

Figure 14: Estrone

synthesized in small amounts by the liver. It helps alleviate vaginal dryness and atrophy and protects against the production of cancer cells. Estriol is the most cancer-protective of the estrogens and is available in the largest quantity, yet it is the least potent estrogen. Estriol has a short half-life and is excreted quickly. It declines first in menopause.

Estriol has been widely used in Europe for more than 50 years. In the United States, however, it isn't widely available, nor does it exist as a prescription medication as estrone and estradiol do. It is available, however, by prescription through compounding pharmacists. Estriol use has grown substantially in the United States over the past 25 years, often combined with bioidentical estrone and estradiol in appropriate ratios in a compounded medication commonly known as Triest.

It is important to ensure that these three estrogens are replaced in proper balance. Some compounded prescriptions might only include E2 and E3 because the body converts E2 into E1. If E2 is metabolized properly, it will provide all the E1 a woman needs. Other women do better with a formulation that contains all three estrogens.

Testing

The only way to really determine hormone levels is through monitoring. In my practice, I use 24-hour urine-hormone levels. They are optimal for monitoring women on HRT, because they measure E1, E2, and E3 along with their metabolites 2,4, and 16 hydroxyestrone. This assures the patient and the doctor that the HRT being prescribed is metabolized into a safe ratio of carcinogenic/noncarcinogenic metabolites.

Saliva testing is also valuable to some extent. However, while it measures free, unbound hormones, such readings are often inaccurate, as certain hormones, such as progesterone, are present in higher levels in the mouth. Patients who take liquid suspensions or lozenges can't be measured accurately through saliva testing. It also doesn't evaluate estrogen metabolites.

Please check the resource section of this book for a summary of the 24-hour urine testing I use in my own practice.

In certain circumstances, serum levels of hormones are more valuable then 24-hour urinary metabolites or can be used in combination with 24-hour urinary hormones. Panels are available that include serum estrone, estradiol, estriol, 2 and 4 hydroxyestrone, progesterone, sex-hormone-binding globulin, DHEA sulphate, and testosterone at affordable pricing.

To assure that the risks of hormone therapy are minimized while being as effective as possible, I think physicians ought to be following some basic guidelines. Please feel free to share this information with your doctor.

(1) Use biologically identical hormones that exactly duplicate the molecular structures of naturally occurring hormones. Drug companies, in order to patent hormones, have altered this molecular structure, causing an altering of the hormone messages received by the cells when these manipulated hormones bind the target-cell-receptor sites. Therefore, most physicians have prescribed and researched hormones that are not biologically identical to hormones the body produces naturally.

(2) Individualize the dose of hormones prescribed for each patient with follow-up lab tests to ensure that the dose is optimal and that the metabolites of hormones like estrogen are not causing any medical risks. (High 4 and 16 hydroxyestrone

might be seen as increasing one's cancer risk, for example.)

(3) Balance all hormones throughout the endocrine system.

(4) Monitor the hormonal balance and metabolism of prescribed hormones rather than giving just estrogen or progesterone. This requires testing the patient for all hormone levels before and after the administration of any HRT. Lab tests to consider include a 24-hour urinary-hormone or serum assay for all male, female, and adrenal hormones and their metabolites, IGF1 levels test (to monitor growth hormone), glucose and insulin levels at 12 hour fasting and one and two hours after drinking 75 grams of glucose and a TSH as a thyroid screening test in combination with temperature charting and a review of possible hypothyroid symptoms. Examples of possible functional thyroid-related symptoms include the following:

▸ chilliness and chronically low body temperatures

▸ waking up tired in the morning (adrenal and thyroid), afternoon fatigue (more thyroid then adrenal)

▶ general lethargy and fatigue, feeling sluggish

▶ an inability to lose weight in spite of caloric restriction (This can be due to too much insulin and/or cortisol or a lack of DHEA, testosterone, and/or growth hormone as well.)

▶ fluid retention

▶ dry skin, hair, or nails

▶ brittle and/or unhealthy nails

▶ hair loss

▶ a low voice

▶ concentration impairment

▶ a tendency toward constipation

▶ slowed reflexes

▶ an enlarged tongue

▶ blood clotting (Thyroid hormone thins the blood.)

▶ high cholesterol (Thyroid hormone lowers one's cholesterol level.)

Other associated symptoms that might improve with thyroid replacement include headaches, insomnia, irritability, anxiety and/or panic, depression, PMS, irregular menstrual cycles, low sexual desire, and low self-esteem. If hypothyroidism is suspected be advised that more comprehensive thyroid assessment and monitoring panels are available, including TSH, Free T4, Free T3, Reverse T3, Antithyroglobulin antibody, and antithyroidalperoxidase antibody.

(5) In the last 10 years the integration of nutritional science with the study of prescription-drug side effects has identified a considerable amount of drug-induced nutrient depletions. Research has shown that estrogen and progesterone replacement can cause folic-acid depletion and increase the risk of cervical dysplasia (precancerous changes of the vaginal cervix). In order to protect nutrient deficiencies caused by hormone replacement therapy, you should supplement not only with folic acid but also with other nutrients, such as, for example, other B vitamins, calcium and magnesium, and minerals. In general, it is a good practice when taking hormone replacement medication of any kind to take a good multivitamin and mineral supplement with at least 800 mcg of folic acid, a total B complex of at least 50 mg, 1,000 mg of calcium, and 500 mg of magnesium. This type of general

supplementation will protect against nutrient depletion. Although currently published studies are on nutrient depletion from conventional manufactured forms of estrogen and synthetic progesterone, some of these same nutrient-depletion interactions may very well occur with customized natural Biest or Triest and with natural progesterone as well.

(6) Protect against the risk of forming clots (thrombi), which have been documented extensively in the literature as a side effect of birth-control pill use and of the synthetic estrogens, premarin and synthetic progesterone (medroxyprogesterone acetate). The risk may or may not be triggered by long-term, normal replacement doses of natural estrogens and progesterone safely metabolized and monitored with testing for blood or urine levels. However, to be on the safe side, I recommend that every 6 to 12 months fibrinogen levels and bleeding times should be monitored. This will reassure both you and your physician that excess fibrin is not accumulating and that platelets aren't clumping or aggregating excessively. The latter development can cause clots in the legs, lungs, heart, and brain as well as

chronic fatigue or fibromyalgia due to a reduced flow of blood and reduced oxygen to the muscles and the brain as well as other tissues. Treatments for blood thinning include high doses of essential fatty acids, as found as in fish oil, flax oil, and borage oil (take 6-10 grams daily), aspirin, and Nattokinase. For more information on Nattokinase I refer you to our website, www.cnm-inc.com, where former papers I have written on Nattokinase and chronic

The Seven Keys to Safe Hormone Replacement Therapy

1. Use bioidentical hormones.
2. Individualize the dose to each person.
3. Monitor the dose with lab testing for all hormones.
4. Balance and test all hormones, not just estrogen and progesterone.
5. Protect against any HRT-induced nutrient deficiencies. Get all your essential nutrients through your diet and through supplementation (amino acids, fatty acids, vitamins, minerals, and trace minerals).
6. Protect against the formation of blood clots.
7. Monitor for other side effects, especially breast tenderness, hair-growth changes, mood swings, and acne.

coagulation are available to download.

It's clear, just prescribing natural estrogen and progesterone is not always the right answer. More often then not, it may be necessary to lower the patient's insulin level by increasing dietary protein, to add DHEA to lower high cortisol level, and/or to help the pituitary secrete more growth hormone as an integrated approach to optimize the patient's health and hormonal equilibrium.

The other important hormones to take are the following:

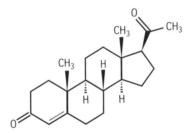

Figure 16: Progesterone

Progesterone:

Often called the "feel-good hormone" due to its antidepressant and mood-enhancing effects, progesterone plays an important role in nervous-system maintenance and helps balance estrogen levels. Taking progesterone with estrogen reduces estrogen dominance and reduces the chances of estrogen-related endometrial cancer and other cancers caused by estrogen. Without adequate natural progesterone, women are at increased risk for uterine fibroids, shortened menstrual cycles, breakthrough bleeding in the middle of the cycle, estrogen dominance, menstrual-cycle migraines, osteoporosis, or excessive estrogen-related weight gain. Progesterone levels naturally rise in the second half of the menstrual cycle to counteract the cell-division and fluid-retention effects of estrogen.

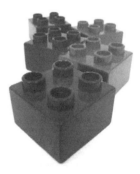

Most fundamentally, progesterone is used as a building-block molecule for many other steroid hormones in the ovaries and adrenals (especially during menopause). Progesterone converts into testosterone, cortisol, and even some estrogen. Furthermore, synthetic molecularly altered progesterone cannot function as a building block for other steroids and can lower the body's production of natural progesterone.

Dehydroepiandrosterone (DHEA):

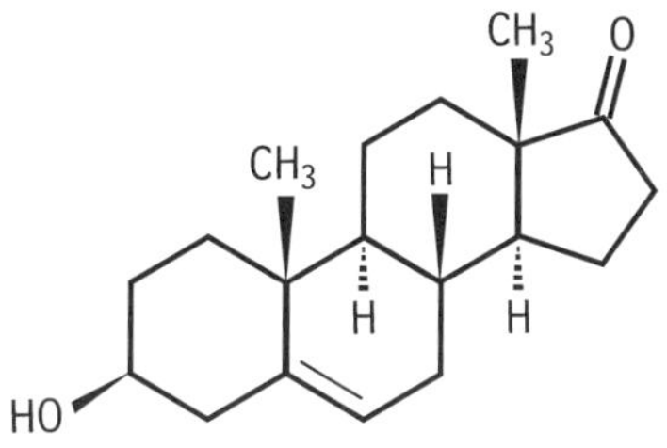

Figure 17: DHEA

DHEA is a steroid hormone that serves as a foundation for the synthesis of other steroid hormones, including estrogen and testosterone. It is the most plentiful anabolic steroid and functions as a precursor to many other muscle- building steroids, including androstenedione and testosterone. If DHEA levels are low, supplements can boost production of these hormones.

Testosterone:

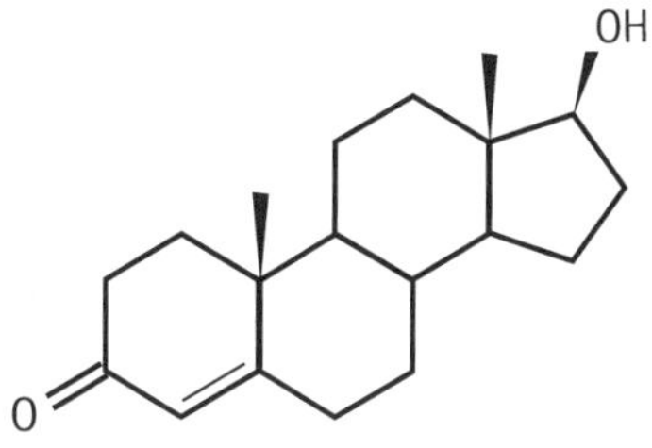

Figure 18: Testosterone

While testosterone is usually considered a male hormone or androgen, women also produce it in smaller amounts. Low levels in women can result in fatigue, depression, joint pain, irritability, osteoporosis, lean-tissue loss, and libido changes.

How Natural Hormones Are Administered

Natural hormones are available in a variety of forms, as a delivery system that works well for one woman may not work as well for another. Everyone absorbs hormones a little differently and responds differently to a given dose. Because of this, you might have to try two or three different forms before you find the one that works best for you.

The most commonly prescribed delivery forms are the following:

▸ **Capsules.** Powder capsules can be formulated for immediate or slow release. Oil capsules can improve the absorption of some hormones—especially progesterone, which is very fat-soluble.

▸ **Sublingual tablets (troche) or liquid suspensions.** Compounds in this form are dissolved under the tongue. The physician can have compounded progesterone, testosterone, DHEA, estradiol, estriol, estrone, biest, triest, or pregnenolone either singly or in combination. Sublingual suspensions have the benefit of enhancing absorption through the sublingual veins and oral mucosa directly into the bloodstream by passing the gut and the first pass of liver metabolism. The dose with this delivery system is usually less than its oral equivalent.

▸ **Creams and ointments.** These delivery forms can be compounded with a variety of different hormones and offer great strength and dosage flexibility. Creams are often absorbed well if the concentration is not compounded too high. Transdermal delivery that is absorbed directly

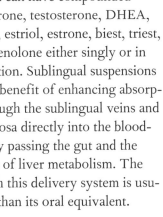

through the skin is beneficial because it is stored in fat cells as a reservoir that gradually accumulates until it forms a steady state of release into the blood and tissues. Transdermal delivery also bypasses the liver and instead metabolizes the hormones on their first pass through the gut, as is the case with oral capsules. Topical creams are also a good choice for women with dry skin. They require application one to three times per day.

▸ Other, less-utilized forms are **suppositories and nasal sprays**.

Estrogens are typically compounded to reflect their natural circulating levels in the body, which are as follows:

▸ 10% to 20% estrone

▸ 10% to 20% estradiol

▸ 60% to 80% estriol

As such, estrogen is often dispensed in precompounded combinations. Biest is usually a combination of estradiol and estriol, commonly in a 20:80 ratio. (Remember that estrone does the same things as estradiol does in the body and both essentially become the same once digested. For women who metabolize estradiol well, not taking additional estrone works fine.) Triest is a combination of all three estrogens in a 10:10:80 ratio of estrone, estradiol, and estriol. Doctors might alter this ratio to 20:20:60 or remove E1 if excessive levels of E1 accumulate. Of the two formulations, Biest has a stronger effect, but many doctors, and I include myself, prefer to replace all three circulating hormones rather than depend on a woman's metabolism to cover one of them.

The average dose of Triest is 2.5 mg. But higher doses can be prescribed, and these ratios can also be changed if symptoms persist. Depending upon the delivery system prescribed and dispensed by the compounding pharmacist (capsule, cream, gel, sublingual liquid suspension, lozenge/troche, or suppository), dosages will vary. Doses should be adjusted according to different absorption rates among individuals. (With Triest at a 1/1/8 ratio, 2.5 mg total volume delivers estrone: 0.25 mg, estradiol: 0.25 mg and estriol: 2 mg. (With Biest at a 2/8 ratio, 2.5 mg. total volume delivers estradiol: 0.5 mg and estriol: 2 mg.)

It is important to realize that even natural, bio-identical hormones can be poorly metabolized. For example oral estradiol (E2) taken in pill form, even when it is natural and bioiden-

tical, gets metabolized through its first pass in the liver and many individuals convert E2 into excessive amount of carcinogenic 16 hydroxy estrone. If physicians don't monitor patients for these metabolites they will not find the patients who are at higher cancer risk.

Furthermore, oral estrogen causes the liver to produce more sex hormone binding globulin (SHBG). This SHBG binds up testosterone and making it less available as free testosterone in the blood. The result can be low levels of testosterone. Interestingly these low levels of testosterone can lead to symptoms that mimic common menopausal complaints including night sweats and hot flashes in women whose estradiol levels still appear normal. This can leave a physician who is not monitoring testosterone levels and SHBG levels perplexed as to why the hot flashes persist when estradiol levels are found to be normal.

Natural progesterone should always be prescribed when estrogen is taken. Dosages here range from 20 to 200 mg during menopause and usually drop to 25 to 50 mg after menopause. Again, this varies depending upon the delivery system used and individual absorption variability.

There are over-the-counter formulations of DHEA available, but they can vary widely in efficacy and strength. For this reason, it's better to take prescription USP (United States Pharmacopia) grade DHEA. Dosages range from 5 to 30 mg daily. It's important to keep an eye on DHEA levels, as excess DHEA will drive cortisol reserves down below normal. DHEA also converts into testosterone. Many postmenopausal women can avoid testosterone replacement and lower high cortisol levels with the correct dosage of DHEA.

Testosterone is typically prescribed for women who don't metabolize enough of it from DHEA. It's given in doses that are one-tenth those used in men—0.5 to 10 mg daily—in order to avoid unwanted side effects. Because it's not effective when taken orally, this hormone is usually prescribed as a topical cream or gel or as a sublingual tablet.

Human growth hormone (HGH) is another hormone women should consider taking. Anyone who has been comprehensively screened for hormone imbalances and is over the age of 40 with confirmed low DHEA may very well have a growth-hormone and related insulin-growth-factor-1 deficiency. The benefits of increasing growth hormone are far-reaching and can include the following:

▶ excellent weight loss

▶ an 8.8% average increase in muscle mass after six months

▶ higher energy levels and increased exercise performance

▶ enhanced sexual performance in men and women

▶ regeneration of the heart, spleen, liver, and kidneys, as well as other organs

▶ better cardiac output plus superior immune and kidney function

▶ lowered blood pressure and an improved cholesterol profile

▶ younger, thicker skin, wrinkle removal and cellulite reduction

▶ hair regrowth

▶ sharper vision

▶ mood elevation

▶ increased memory retention

▶ improved sleep

To Cycle or Not to Cycle

Women's sex hormones are sent from and received by the ovaries in a recurring pattern. Hormone receptors are accustomed to the pattern, so it may be beneficial to take hormones in cycles as follows:

- ▸ estrogen—first three weeks

- ▸ progesterone—weeks three and four

- ▸ testosterone—weeks one through three

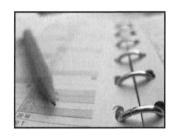

- ▸ DHEA— throughout the month (every day)

There are, however, potential problems with this therapy, despite its appearance of being consistent with a woman's natural cyclic patterns, such as, for example, the following:

- ▸ Some women may find it difficult to follow with different hormones being taken each week. While this can be simplified with blister-pack weekly dosing packets, the cost of therapy goes up significantly.

- ▸ This type of dosing tends to build up the endometrial lining and then reduce it by estrogen withdrawal. This can lead to breakthrough menstrual bleeding in menopausal women. Many women prefer to leave their menstruation behind. There is clinical evidence accumulated over years of study that continuous, even daily, dosing keeps the uterine walls inactive without risking excessive endometrial build-up.

- ▸ There is a greater chance of getting estrogen-withdrawal symptoms, such as hot flashes, night sweats, and mood changes returning in the fourth week each month.

How You Can Get Natural Hormones

Finding someone to prescribe natural hormones is getting easier as more health-care professionals realize the importance of tailoring medications to meet individual needs. That said, it could still be somewhat difficult to tap into the resources you need to obtain natural-hormone therapy. While natural hormones are not subject to FDA regulation and don't have to go through the safety-and-efficacy trials required of other drugs, you will still need a prescription from a medical doctor, nurse practitioner, or naturopathic physician for estrogens and testosterone. Progesterone and DHEA are available in over-the-counter formulations, but they're best obtained by prescription as well.

The second factor that can affect your ability to obtain natural hormones is the availability of a compounding pharmacy in your area. The good news is that while there were no more than a few hundred of these specialty pharmacies in the United States in the 1970s, there are now well over 4,000 of them across the country. Although they're not available everywhere, a number of them now do a thriving mail-order business.

Several resources for locating physicians who prescribe natural hormones and pharmacies that compound them can be found in the resources section at the back of the book.

No Matter What You Are Taking, Commit to Being Monitored.

It takes three months and sometimes longer for hormones, especially steroids, taken orally or transdermally (through the skin) to reach a steady level in the bloodstream and to bind consistently to fat cells. It is essential to monitor hormone levels every three to six months until your dose is stable and you feel good.

I recommend that if at all possible you initially utilize 24-hour urine or serum panels so dosages can be adjusted accordingly. Remember that these are potent hormones and that diligent monitoring that evaluates metabolic safety as well as effectiveness of the therapy is very important. Taking 24-hour urine levels is so valuable because your hormones are released in a pulsed fashion throughout the day and this kind of monitoring averages those pulses into a predictable level in the urine. It is the gold standard for cortisol levels, and it is the only way to effectively assess estrogen-related metabolism cancer risk.

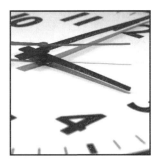

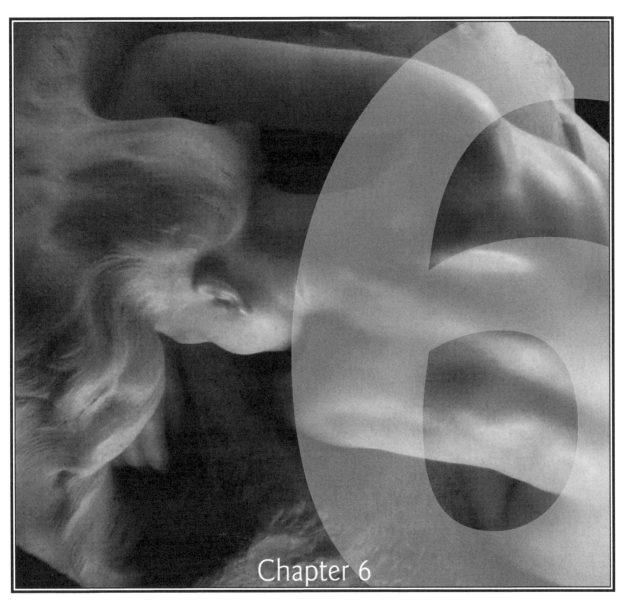

Chapter 6

From Biochemical Individuality to
Genetic Individuality

Chapter 6

From Biochemical Individuality to Genetic Individuality

In 1956 a book called <u>Biochemical Individuality</u> by Roger Williams, Ph.D. dramatically changed our perspective on the relationship between nutritional needs and the individual. Biochemical individuality, a somewhat intimidating term, simply is the theory that because individuals have different lifestyles and stressors they create different levels of nutritional needs. In other words, no two people have the exact same nutritional needs.

Before Roger Williams published <u>Biochemical Individuality</u> the average nutritionist believed that everyone could achieve optimal health as long as they were receiving the recommended daily allowances for calories, protein, fats, carbohydrates, fiber, vitamins, minerals and trace minerals. However, these days we recognize that an athlete sweating profusely on a basketball court for two hours a day, seven days a week will lose more electrolytes, minerals, and water stores and has greater caloric needs than a couch potato. The individual who smokes one to two packs of cigarettes a day needs more essential fatty acids to prevent the thickening of blood caused by tobacco smoke (smokers almost always have high fibrinogen levels and excess fibrin strands in their blood). The same smoker also needs much higher levels of antioxidants than her non-smoking counterpart. The woman who eats heated oxidized saturated fat on a daily bases from animal sources also has greater antioxidant needs than her vegetarian friend. The vegetarian on the other hand needs to be careful to avoid a deficiency in protein, B vitamin, or essential fatty acid.

Other individuals may develop abnormal intestinal flora, food allergies or an intestinal malabsorption from gluten sensitivity or a leaky intestinal wall lining. Intestinal abnormalities like these can often remain hidden and undiagnosed creating the need for a greater amount of nutrients in order to guarantee optimal nutrition into the cells until the gut lining is healed.

These are all examples of biochemical individuality. There are many more. In fact every chronic disease from diabetes to arthritis, from allergies to hypertension, causes an individual's nutritional needs to be unique. Certain drugs can lead to nutritional deficiencies creating a need for higher doses of certain B vitamins, minerals, and other nutrients such as coenzyme Q-10 and alpha lipoic acid.

Clinical nutrition has increased in its sophistication to the point where one's biochemical individuality can be more accurately determined. Tests are now available that can look for deficiencies in vitamins, minerals and essential fatty acids. Any nutritionally oriented physician will be able to guide you in the proper selection of the most valuable tests for you to consider.

Completed in 2003, the Human Genome Project (HGP) was a 13-year project coordinated by the U.S. Department of Energy and

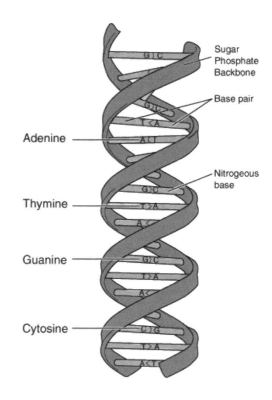

Figure 19: Structure of DNA

the National Institutes of Health. The HGP's goals where to:

- *identify* all the approximately 20,000-25,000 genes in human DNA within the 23 paired chromosomes inherited from one's parents

- *determine* the sequences of the 3 billion chemical base pairs that make up human DNA

▶ *store* this information in databases

▶ *improve* tools for data analysis

▶ *transfer* related technologies to the private sector and

▶ *address* the ethical, legal, and social issues (ELSI) that may arise from the project

At birth you inherit two sets of genes—one set from each of your parents. Each gene contains a set of coded instructions that "explain" to your body how it will develop and function. Your height, your eye color, your voice, your hair texture—even certain elements of your personality—are strongly influenced by your genes.

Genes contain long double-stranded segments called DNA (deoxyribonucleic acid). DNA is formed by a sequence of four chemicals (called nucleotides). The arrangement of these four nucleotides, acting like rungs on a ladder, makes up your genetic code. No two individuals (except identical twins) are born with the same exact arrangement. In fact, just by changing the order of these four chemicals, all the wondrous genetic diversity within the human race is created.

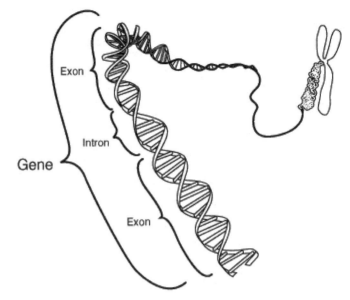

Figure 20: A Gene

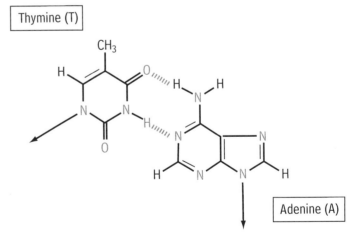

Figure 21: A nucleotide pair

With the successful mapping of the entire DNA code came the understanding that many individuals are born with slight alternations in their genetic code. One single rung on the ladder that should have been formed by the nucleotides adenine paired with thymine and guanine paired with cytosine (see Figures 21 and 22) end up being paired in a different sequence than the typical human genome.

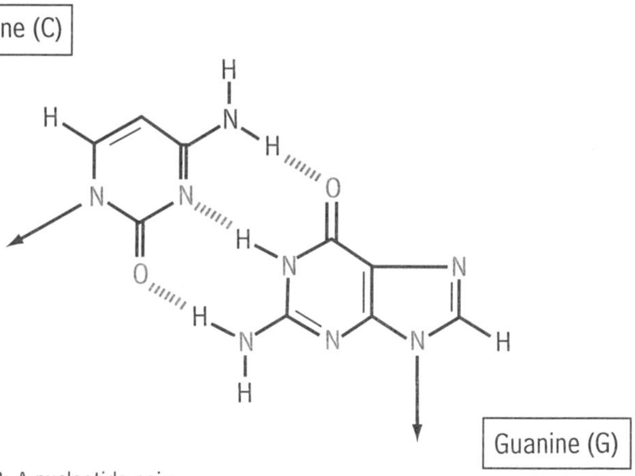

Figure 22: A nucleotide pair

Using cells collected either from a simple mouth rinse procedure or from a single blood draw, genetic tests measure selected segments of the genetic code that differ from individual to individual. These are called single nucleotide polymorphisms, or SNPs for short.

SNPs are variations in the genetic code that occur only at certain places, in certain individuals. These SNPs serve as substitutes of the nucleotides that typically create the ladder rungs of the DNA code. Everyone has SNPs—that's what makes us different from one another. Some SNPs are quite common and others are quite rare. Many SNPs have no effect on our health, but others can predispose us to disease or influence our response to a food or drug.

Even SNPs that are good for our health in one situation may be harmful in another. For example, the same SNP that enables a person to better survive on a very limited food intake in situations of starvation, may cause that person to be more prone to obesity and cholesterol build-up in the blood after eating fatty foods.

It's very important to remember that the SNPs included in genetic testing indicate risk, not certainty. Testing positive for a SNP doesn't mean you are sure to develop a health problem. By the same token, if you don't have a SNP associated with a certain disease, that doesn't mean you are completely protected from that disease, or that you shouldn't take steps to optimize your health. It just means that your genetic risk is lower for that disease.

In the past the idea of genetic testing was often met with resistance by the general public. People questioned why they should bother with testing since the perception was that they couldn't do anything about what they had inherited anyway. These days, nothing could

be further from the truth. For example, in the cutting edge field of genomic nutrition, a woman with a methylenetetrahydrofolate reductase single nucleotide polymorphism is recognized as having a genetic individuality that requires her to take larger amounts of certain nutrients to combat elevated homocysteine levels and vasoconstricting elements that can lead to cardiovascular disease. (See the sidebar for more information on these specific nutrients.)

How does genetic testing relate to menopause? As it turns out several relatively common SNPs can have significant effects on the metabolism of estrogen. For example, a relatively common SNP affecting estrogen metabolism is a SNP on the COMT (catechol-O-methyl transferase enzyme) gene in position V158M on the human genome. This COMT enzyme is primarily responsible for the breaking down of neurotransmitters including dopamine, norepinephrine, epinephrine, as well as the methylating of estradiol for safe removal as well as the safe removal via methylation of carcinogenic 4-hydroxyestrone. When these neurotransmitters are not effectively broken down the build up can lead to anti-social behavior, violence and in some cases even schizophrenia. COMT also plays

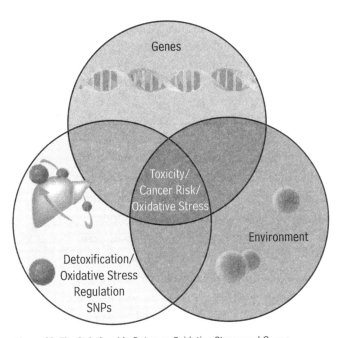

Figure 23: The Relationship Between Oxidative Stress and Genes
(Picture and information used with permission from Great Smokies Diagnostic Laboratory and Genovations.)

the important roles of converting 2-hydroxye-strogens into compounds with anti-carcino-genic properties and inhibiting the prolifera-tion of human breast cancer cells. A SNP at this same location has also been associated with carcinogenic estrogen metabolism, depression, ADHD (attention deficit disor-der), alcoholism, and bipolar disorders.

Increasing the amount of methylating support nutrients a woman with this particular SNP gets would help to optimize her health. This is especially essential for any woman taking any form of estrogen replacement ther-apy, for individuals with cancer risk, or for women who have this SNP and suffer from depression, ADHD, or bipolar disorder.

The last SNP associated with estrogen embolism is CYP1B1 one of the cytochrome P 450 phase 1 liver detoxification enzymes. CYP1B1 is specifically involved with the deactivation and the safe metabolism of a rela-tively potent free radical metabolite of estradi-ol and estrone called 4 hydroxyestrone. This CYP1B1 enzyme is specifically found in breast, ovary, prostate and kidney tissues rather than liver tissue. Individuals with this SNP accumulate excessive amounts of 4 hydroxyestrone and as a result have less of the more cancer protective 2 hydroxyestrone on

The nutrients that may be used to fight a pre-disposition to cardiovascular dis-ease include the amino acid methionine and s adenyl methionine (SAMe) in combination with folic acid (especially in its active form of L-5-methyl tetrahydrofolate), riboflavin, vitamin B_{12} (ideally in the form of methyl-cobalamin), vitamin B_6 (ideally in its active form of pyridoxyl 5 phosphate), vitamin B_2 riboflavin, trimethylglycine and choline. Formulas available at the Center for Natural Medicine Mail Order Dispensary (www.cnm-inc.com) include Vessel Care by Metagenics, Coenzymate B Complex by Source Naturals, and SAM-e Plus by Karuna. See the resource section at the end at the end of the book.

board. Again increasing the amount of methy-lating nutrients is called for in these cases as well adding more foods to the diet that aid phase 1 liver detoxification. These foods include fruits and vegetables (especially cru-ciferous vegetables like broccoli, Brussels sprouts, cauliflower, watercress and cabbage) along with, green and black teas, and a variety of herbs including rosemary, basil, turmeric, cumin, poppy seeds and black pepper.

It is interesting to note that in most cases,

a gene's ability to promote disease depends in large measure on the gene being switched "on" or "off" by factors in the environment. Examples of environmental factors that can switch a gene's expression to the promotion of disease include air pollution, cigarette smoking, poor diet, excessive alcohol or drug intake, infections, hormone imbalances, nutrient deficiencies, heavy metal toxicity and lifestyle/emotional stress.

The majority of genetic polymorphisms have the potential rather than the genetic guarantee to cause health problems. Knowing these genetic variations exist and adjusting your lifestyle and supplementation accordingly can help prevent ever developing certain health problems or more adequately supporting these health problems once they develop. With targeted optimal nutrition necessary you can overcome genetic weaknesses. With the unraveling of the human genome comes a new frontier of genomic nutrition where your individual genetic uniqueness can be identified and this information can be used to customize your diet and supplementation in a way that supports your genetic weaknesses while maximizing your genetic potential.

While genomic profiling is a cutting edge idea there are several labs already offering this breakthrough in individualized care. You'll find contact information for one that I recommend, Great Smokies, in the resource section at the back of this book.

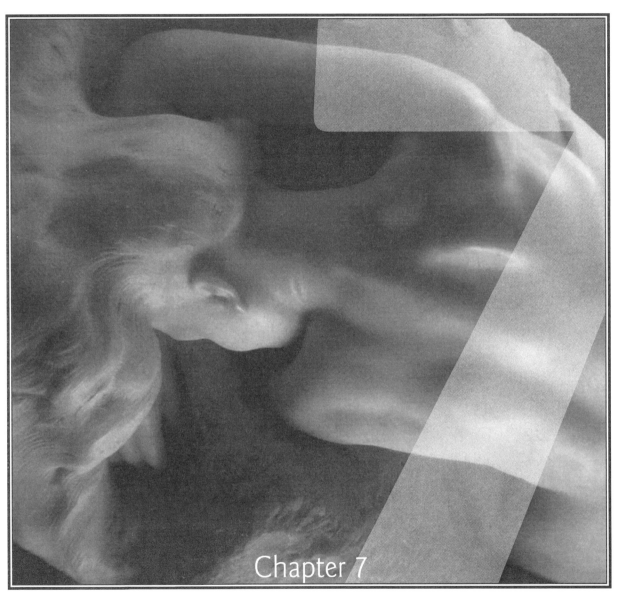

Chapter 7

Eating for Life

Chapter 7
Eating for Life

In the collection of tools that can be used to fight the negative symptoms associated with menopause, nutrition has traditionally taken a back seat. But no more. Thanks to ongoing nutritional research, and research that focuses specifically on the nutritional needs of women, we now know that certain foods can have a significant effect on how women experience menopause. A well-balanced diet, one that supplies the right kinds of nutrients and the proper amounts of them, can play a key role in easing some of the symptoms of menopause and ensuring better health in the years ahead.

By the time they reach their menopausal years, however, many women find themselves uncertain about what exactly constitutes a healthy diet and, specifically, what they should be eating to support their good health, both during menopause and after it. This is understandable, especially given the conflicting opinions that seem to arise almost daily about what constitutes healthy eating. One study will espouse the benefits of alcohol consumption, while another will knock it down. It's enough to make your head spin, regardless of who you are and what your specific health issues might be.

This chapter will help you sort through the sea of conflicting information that's out there. While food may at times seem more like a foe than a friend, it's important to know that some of the most powerful menopause-symptom fighters are—or can be—no farther away than your pantry or refrigerator.

In the whole-body approach to treating menopause, nutrition is one of the most important factors. Many of the physical and emotional issues that often accompany menopause, such as mood swings, weight gain, and depression, are attributed to the hormonal shifts that take place during menopause. However, food can also play an important role. Just making some simple dietary changes can make a significant difference in easing the transition through menopause.

Phytoestrogens, which are naturally occurring plant compounds that can produce estrogenic effects, often garner the lion's share of attention when nutrition for the menopausal years is discussed. I'll spend some time discussing them here as well. First, however, let's take a closer look at why the food we eat plays such a big role in how we feel. Along the way, you'll also learn more about why the carbohydrate-laden eating plans that so many women follow can actually make your menopause symptoms get worse.

Food, Glorious Food

Although we rarely, if ever, stop to consider it as such, food is one of the most potent drugs known to mankind. Comprised of macronutrients—proteins, carbohydrates, and fats—and micronutrients—vitamins and minerals—the food you eat has a tremendous effect on both your physical and mental health.

To understand the specific actions that food has on the body, let's take a quick look at the macronutrients and what they do. I'll discuss the micronutrients further in Chapter 8.

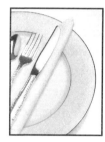

Protein Power

Protein has received a fair amount of bad press in recent years, largely due to the high-protein/high-carb diet debate and concerns that consuming too much protein can be bad for your health. While protein has its detractors, there is no denying the essential role it plays in the body. Adequate protein intake is essential for tissue growth, repair, and maintenance. Protein also plays a key role in the immune system, helps makes hormones, and carries nutrients throughout the body.

For menopausal women, adequate protein intake is essential for keeping blood-sugar levels stable. Protein turns into sugar more slowly than do carbohydrates and fats. Unfortunately, many women tend to avoid this important macronutrient because of their mostly unfounded concerns about protein's effect on their weight. At four kilocalories per gram—the same amount as carbohydrates contain—protein itself is not the culprit when it comes to weight control. Portion size and the fat that often comes along with protein are more to blame, as I'll explain in more detail later.

Protein is comprised of more than 20 amino acids. Your body can make the majority of the amino acids it needs, but not all of them. The 11 amino acids manufactured by the body are called nonessential because they don't have to come from outside sources. For humans, there are nine essential amino acids that must be supplied by the diet. Some authors have extended this list to 12 essential amino acids, including several that although they can be synthesized in the body are often manufactured in inadequate amounts, such as, for example, taurine.

When you consume protein your body breaks down the amino acids and combines them with the ones your body already produces, creating new proteins for growth, repair, and other bodily functions. If you are

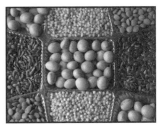

not getting enough energy from other macronutrients in your diet, your body will also use the protein you consume as a source of energy. The more protein your body uses for creating energy, the less there is available for the body to draw the essential amino acids from. Without adequate amounts of these essential amino acids, your body may not be able to perform certain important functions, which could potentially, lead to health problems.

Animal vs. Vegetable Protein

Both animals and plants make protein out of amino acids. Plants do this by combining simple sugars with nitrogen from the air and soil. Each plant makes proteins that are unique to it; however, plants manufacture incomplete proteins that don't contain all the amino acids

If you rely on plant proteins as your primary protein source, it's necessary to eat a wide variety of them to provide the body with the amino acids it requires to meet its protein needs. Two essential amino acids, lysine and tryptophan, are poorly represented in most plant proteins, so vegetarians should be particularly careful to make sure they have enough of both in their diet.

that the human body needs. Grains and legumes, for example, lack lysine but contain methionine. Because animals both eat foods that contain amino acids and manufacture their own, animal protein is generally considered a complete protein that contains all the amino acids the body needs.

Plant Protein

Most plant proteins aren't high in fat, so

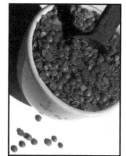

you don't have to worry about it as much when you eat them. What is important is choosing the plant sources that have the most protein, such as tofu, soybeans, legumes, and beans, so you don't have to eat large quantities of them to meet your nutritional needs.

Table 5: Vegetable-protein Sources

Vegetable-protein Sources	Protein (grams)	Vegetable-protein Sources	Protein (grams)	Vegetable-protein Sources	Protein (grams)
soy burger	18	soy hotdog	8	cashews (1 oz.)	5
spirulina powder* (1 oz.)	16	split peas	8	rice, brown (1 cup)	5
tofu (6 oz.)	12	soy milk (1 cup)	7	sesame seeds (1 oz.)	5
soybeans	11	pasta (1 cup)	7	almonds (1 oz.)	5
chickpeas	10	chili beans	7	green peas	4
hummus (chickpea spread)	10	black-eyed peas	7	soy sausages (one link)	4
lentils	9	garbanzo beans	7	potato, baked (small)	3
kidney beans	8	flaxseed (1 oz.)	6	rice, white (1 cup)	3
navy beans	8	sunflower seeds (1 oz.)	6	spinach	2
peanuts (1 oz.)	8	butter beans	6	broccoli	2
peanut butter (2 TB.)	8	lima beans	6	corn	2
pinto beans	8	oatmeal (1 cup)	6	green beans	2
white beans	8	bread, whole wheat (2 slices)	5	squash	1

(All serving sizes are 1/2 cup unless otherwise noted.)

* dried seaweed

Animal Protein

Animal protein often gets a bad rap for being high in fat, but the truth is that not all of it is that bad. You simply need to be more choosy about what animal proteins you eat. The foods listed here provide all the good things that protein has going for it without being high in fat.

When you choose source of animal protein, it's a good idea to select products that are as unadulterated or pure as possible. Many animals raised for com- mercial-food purposes are treated with hormones or hormonally related products to promote growth or increase the yield. While studies are inconclusive, a growing number of experts believe that people who eat products from hormone-treated animals are at greater risk of developing hormonally related cancers. In fact, two studies reported upon in fall 2002 found that dairy

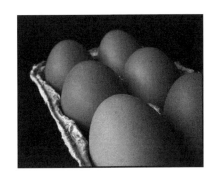

Table 6: Animal-protein Sources

Animal-protein Sources	Protein (grams)	Animal-protein Sources	Protein (grams)	Animal-protein Sources	Protein (grams)
protein bars	32 to 8*	Canadian bacon	21	crab	13
cottage cheese, fat-free (1 cup)	30	sardines (canned)	21	yogurt, fat-free or low-fat (1 cup)	10
protein powder	30 to 16*	herring (uncreamed or smoked)	20	milk, skim (1 cup)	8
chicken breast (without skin)	26	salmon	18	cheese, low-cal (1 oz)	7
turkey breast (without skin)	26	ham, canned (lean)	18	egg (1)	6
Tuna, white, canned in water	25	shrimp	17	bacon (1 slice)	5-8
pork tenderloin	21	swordfish	17	luncheon meat, 95% fat-free (1 oz.)	5
beef, lean, (USDA good or choice quality), including sirloin, round, and flank steak	21	beef, hamburger, (cooked)	14	egg white (1)	4
		scallops	14	whey protein from milk (the most concentrated source)	67
buffalo	21	venison	13		

(All serving sizes are 3 ounces unless otherwise indicated.)

* depending on the product

products might raise blood levels of a cancer-promoting hormone in women. However, it still isn't clear whether milk itself, or a particular component of it was to blame.

How Much Protein Is Enough?

If you do some research on recommended daily protein intake you'll find that there are widely varying opinions as to how much is needed. The recommended daily allowance (RDA) established by the U.S. government, calls for 0.8 gram per kilogram (2.2 pounds) of ideal body weight. For a 150-pound woman, this equates to just over 54 grams of protein a day. Nutritionists often go a bit higher and recommend between 0.4 to 0.45 grams of protein per pound of body weight per day, or 60 to 67.5 grams for a 150-pound woman.

The truth is that protein needs can vary quite a bit from person to person, so there really isn't one exact figure to go by. Active individuals need more protein than sedentary people do, typically around 0.15 to 0.35 more per pound. People who are trying to lose weight actually need to eat even more protein, typically between 0.7 and 1.0 total grams per pound. If you have a medical problem that impairs your metabolism, such as hypoglycemia, diabetes, polycystic ovarian syndrome, syndrome X, or high triglycerides in the blood, you need even more protein and less dietary carbohydrates.

While some research has shown that people don't need as much protein as previously thought, more recent studies indicate that women—and especially women who are approaching their menopause years or are in them—need about 1 gram of protein daily per pound of body weight to maintain muscle mass and boost metabolism. Some studies also confirm that eating animal protein does not increase the risk of heart disease, as was once previously thought.

The FDA has approved six different kinds of steroid hormones for use in food production in the United States: estradiol, progesterone, testosterone, zeranol, trenbolone acetate, and melengestrol acetate. Zeranol, trenbolone acetate, and melengesterol acetate are hormone-type chemicals that make animals grow faster. Currently, federal regulations allow these hormones to be used on growing cattle and sheep but not on poultry or hogs.

Still, it's important to keep in mind that it is easy to overdo it when it comes to protein. If animal protein is your primary protein source, you can meet your protein needs very easily by eating relatively small amounts. For example, one 3-oz. serving of chicken breast has 26 grams of protein. Most people eat at least double this size portion in just one sitting. For some women, this one meal can comprise more than 50 percent of their daily protein needs. Switching to plant proteins for at least some of your daily intake will allow you to eat more, so you will feel full and satisfied without going overboard on the protein.

The Dangers of Eating Too Much Protein

Your body knows its protein requirements, and it will only use as much as it needs. If you are very active, the protein you eat but don't use might go to energy, but more often than not it is just extra calories, and they have to go somewhere. That "somewhere" usually translates into extra pounds. Plus, if you're eating animal protein, it's accompanied by fat, another contributor to excess weight and other health concerns.

Diets that are too high in protein can overburden your kidneys. When the body metabolizes protein, ammonia, which is highly toxic to the body, is left behind as a waste product. To protect itself, the body converts ammonia to urea, which, though less toxic, is still something your body needs to eliminate quickly. The kidneys filter urea from the blood and send it to the bladder in the urine. The more urea that your body creates, the harder the kidneys have to work to get rid of it.

Diets that are too high in protein can also lead to the following conditions:

▸ **Ketosis:** Ketosis develops when the diet doesn't contain enough carbohydrates, which are necessary for efficient fat burning. Fats that don't break down correctly develop into acid-like substances called ketone bodies. When these keytone bodies accumulate, they cause an increase in the acidity of the body's fluids via a process called "ketosis" or "acidosis." Symptoms of ketosis include dizziness, nausea, fatigue, confusion, abdominal pain, and bad breath. Some amount of controlled ketosis can be tolerated. In fact, many high-protein diets are designed to place a person in ketosis. The benefit of controlled ketosis is that energy is burned directly from fat rather than from carbohydrates and the person is guaranteed to be losing weight from fat stores. In my practice, when we place people on high-protein diets, we monitor their first morning concentrated urine for ideal ketosis, using a dipstick. An ideal urine dipstick measurement is 15. More ketosis than this can be dangerous. We also encourage drinking plenty of water to make the ketosis easier on the kidneys.

▸ **Osteoporosis:** Calcium, along with other important minerals, is excreted in urine. High-protein diets, which promote fluid loss, can contribute to excess calcium loss. It's also important to note that the calcium, instead of being excreted, can build up in the kidneys, leading to kidney stones. If you are on a high-protein diet, taking more calcium, especially in the form of ionized coral calcium, highly bioavailable liquid calcium or calcium chelates, will help reduce the acidity of the high-protein diet and will add protection against any osteoporosis risk. You can purchase these calcium supplements in some health-food

stores and from a number of Internet sources. See the resource section at the back of this book for information on the calcium product we use at the Center for Natural Medicine Inc.

▸ **Gout:** This painful, arthritic-type condition is caused by uric acid accumulating around joints, tendons, and other body tissues. Foods that are high in purines, such as certain meats, seafood, and some dried beans and peas, metabolize to uric acid in the body. With the supervision of a physician, gout can be controlled naturally with high doses of folic acid (5 mg-30 mg). Folic acid works by blocking xanthine oxidase, which is needed to convert purines into uric acid. Folic acid also lowers homocysteine levels and helps with the recycling of methionine. It is important to note that the birth-control-pill commonly causes a folic-acid deficiency. The high uric-acid levels, which lead to more pain and inflammation, can also be effectively neutralized with ionized, bioavailable calcium. See the resource section at the back of this book for information on how to test the pH (acid-base balance) of your urine and saliva.

Phytoestrogens

Switching to plant proteins has the added benefit of boosting your intake of phytoestrogens, plant-based estrogens that may help curb some of the symptoms associated with menopause, such as hot flashes, and may possibly have beneficial effects on cardiovascular and bone health.

Although phytoestrogens are plant-based, their chemical makeup allows them to bind to estrogen receptors in humans. While they are hundreds to thousands of times weaker than natural estrogen, they can circulate in the blood at significantly higher levels than natural estrogen. Some will also bind to progesterone receptors and act as weak estrogen or estrogen precursors.

There are many different types of phytoestrogens. Of them, isoflavones, coumestans, and lignans are the most commonly studied.

Isoflavones

Isoflavones are the most potent phytoestrogens. There are more than 1,000 different types; of them, genistein and daidzein, which are found in legumes (soy, chickpeas, lentils, clover, and beans), appear to be highest in estrogenic properties.

Soy and soy products contain the highest levels of isoflavones. However, the amount that they contain can vary a great deal. Three ounces of tofu, for example, contains around 23 mg of isoflavones, making it a top choice among the plant proteins. Processed soy products, such as milk and flour, contain lower amounts. Beware when purchasing these processed products. Many have been genetically engineered with an altered seedpod used in the farming. Whenever possible, purchase organic, non-genetically altered soy.

In addition to bestowing estrogenic and antiestrogenic benefits, soy isoflavones act as powerful antioxidants. As such, they may help prevent cancer and enhance immune-system functioning. Soy phytoestrogens in particular have been shown to block estrogen receptors from absorbing excess natural estrogen, possibly preventing some cancers.

Coumestans

Coumestans, which are believed to be 30

to 100 times more potent than isoflavones, are found in the sprouts of some plants, such as alfalfa and certain clovers (both contain the highest amounts of coumestans), as well as in various beans and legumes such as split peas, pinto beans, and lima beans. Coumesterol has been shown to have both estrogenic and anti-estrogenic qualities. By inhibiting estrone-to-estradiol conversion, it may help lower estrogen activity in women with excess estrogen. On the flip side, it can increase sex-hormone-binding globulin (SHBG), which, in turn, increases the availability of estrogens in women with low levels.

Lignans

Lignans are found in higher-fiber foods, such as flaxseed, lentils, whole grains, beans, fruits, and vegetables. In the intestine, lignans are converted into two substances—enterolactone and enterodiol—both of which have estrogen-like effects.

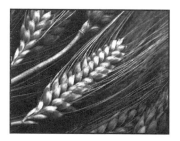

Lignans are being studied for possible use in cancer prevention, particularly breast cancer. They may also be antioxidants and might have a role in lowering cholesterol.

Flaxseed is a phenomenal source of phytoestrogen lignans—in fact, it contains 100 times more lignans than the next highest source. These protective compounds work as estrogen modulators, and studies suggest they may offer protection from hormone-sensitive cancers.

While it's a good idea to add phytoestrogens to your diet, as most people take in far too little of them, it's best not to overdo it. The estrogenic effect they have in humans could lead to an increased breast-cancer risk. This risk has been extensively studied, with conflicting results. Some studies report no link between these products and breast cancer; others have reported a decreased risk for those women who eat soy.

The Lowdown on Fat

We've heard so much about fat's evils that it's hard to believe there is anything good about it. Certainly, eating too much fat, and especially the wrong kinds of fat, can lead to significant health problems, including obesity, heart disease, and cancer. But eating too little fat can also disrupt the body's normal biological functions. The goal is to strike a healthy level of fat intake and by knowing which fats to avoid.

Dietary fat is necessary for the following purposes:

- transporting the fat-soluble vitamins A, D, E, and K (without fat to circulate, store, and absorb these vitamins, the body can't use them.)

- supplying essential fatty acids, such as linoleic acid, gamma linolenic acid, and alpha linolenic acid, that the body can't manufacture

- supporting such vital bodily functions as metabolism and cell growth and repair

Eating a moderate amount of fat also helps us to feel full, as it remains in the stomach longer than carbohydrates and proteins do.

In the body, most fat travels around in the form of fatty acids that couple with a type of glycerol molecule. Glycerol has three carbon atoms, which is what the fatty acids link to. When three fatty acids couple onto a carbon atom, they form a triglyceride—which is the fat that gets stored in fat cells. Triglycerides also make up the majority of fat that circulates in the blood and are the main type of fat found in food, accounting for 98 percent of the fat we eat.

Depending on their chemical composition, there are three types of triglycerides:

- Saturated fats. These fats carry as many hydrogen atoms as chemically possible. They are the most dangerous kind of fat and are the leading contributor to high blood-cholesterol levels and to heart disease. Saturated fats are solid at room temperature and primarily come from animal sources.

- Monounsaturated fats. These fats are not completely saturated with hydrogen atoms. Studies have shown that monounsaturated fats can actually help lower blood-cholesterol levels. They are liquid at room temperature and come from plant sources.

▶ Polyunsaturated fats. Fats in this category have two or more double carbon bonds, which means that they are even less saturated than monounsaturated fats. Fats in this category, especially those found in fish, have been proven to reduce the risk of heart disease. They, too, are liquid at room temperature.

Vegetable oils that have been changed into semisolid form through hydrogenation, such as lard substitutes and tub and stick margarine, contain what are called transfatty acids. They make these altered vegetable oils act more like saturated fat in the body, which means they can also raise blood-cholesterol levels. Some studies also point to higher incidences of breast cancer among women who use these products. Research also shows that transfatty acids might also interfere with the body's natural manufacturing of hormones. A study of nearly 800 post-menopausal European women showed that those whose bodies contained the highest levels of transfatty acids were 40 percent more likely to develop breast cancer than those with the lowest levels.

In 2003, the U.S. Food and Drug Administration amended its regulations on nutrition labeling to require that transfatty acids be disclosed on a separate line immediately under the line for the declaration of saturated fatty acids. Firms were given more than a year to implement the labeling changes, which are scheduled to go into effect on January 1, 2006.

When it comes to protecting your heart

> All food that contains fat consists of both saturated and unsaturated fatty acids, mixed together in different proportions. Butter, for example, contains about 65 percent saturated fatty acids. Coconut oil is even higher at 91 percent. Olive oil is high on the monounsaturated-fatty-acids list at 77 percent.

Table 7: Types of Fat

Saturated	Monounsaturated	Polyunsaturated
animal fat	almond oil	corn oil
butter fat	canola oil	cottonseed oil
coconut oil	olive oil	fish oil
palm kernel oil	peanut oil	flaxseed oil
palm oil		grapeseed oil
		safflower oil
		sesame oil
		soybean oil
		sunflower oil
		walnut oil

health, plant-derived fats are still a better choice than animal fats. If you're going to use them in solid form, be sure to choose those that are labeled as having no transfatty acids. Also limit your exposure to transfatty acids by avoiding processed baked goods, which often contain high levels of them.

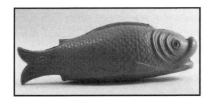

Omega Oils—Essential Fatty Acids

In recent years, studies have shown that certain types of fatty acids can actually contribute to good health. Known as omega-3s, these fats are found primarily in the oils of cold-water fish, shellfish, and sea mammals.

Fish oil has proven to be so beneficial to heart health that the American Heart Association now recommends eating oily, cold-water fish like tuna, herring, sardines, and mackerel on a regular basis—at least once or twice a week. If, for some reason you prefer to not eat fish, another great option is taking fish-oil supplements daily. If you like fish

and choose to add more of it to your diet, be advised that tuna has been found to be a high source of mercury contamination.

Omega-3s can also be found in varying degrees in some nuts and seeds, such as flaxseed, hemp seed, soybeans, and walnuts, as well as the oils derived from them. You can add omega-3s to your diet by eating dark, leafy vegetables. You can also buy special eggs that have high omega-3 levels, which come from chickens that eat algae along with their chicken feed.

Omega-6 is another omega fat that should be a part of your healthy diet. It's an important source of linoleic acid, an essential fatty

A good way to boost your omega-3 and fiber intake is to purchase organic flaxseeds and grind them fresh each morning in a coffee-bean grinder for a full 20-30 seconds until a fine powder is formed. Then add 2-4 tablespoons into a morning smoothie with frozen organic berries, soy milk, and/or whey protein. Adjust the amount of ground-flax until your stools are about as wide as the circle formed by your thumb and index finger. This will mean that you are getting enough fiber in your diet. Flax, taken ground in this form not only is a great source of fiber but also contains cancer-protective lignans and is a great source of essential fatty acids, both omega 3 and omega 6.

acid that is also vital to good health. Omega-6 is contained in many seeds and a number of vegetable oils, including corn, grapeseed, peanut, soybean, and sunflower. Evening primrose is an especially good source of Omega-6. It's also found in the fat of animals that are raised on corn.

Concerning Cholesterol

Cholesterol is the precursor for steroid hormones, which means that it's essential for sustaining life. This hard, waxy, fatlike substance can be found in all parts of the body, including the nervous system, muscles, skin, liver, intestines, and heart. The liver produces all the cholesterol the body needs. Even if you never ate any foods that contain cholesterol, you'd still have some in your body.

Like fat, cholesterol has been highly publicized for its role in promoting heart disease. And, just as with fat, the vital role it plays in the body is also largely overshadowed because of it. In addition to enabling the formation of sex hormones, cholesterol also does the following important tasks:

▸ forms and maintains cell membranes

▸ assists the production of bile salts, which help to digest food

▸ assists in the synthesis of vitamin D

Plant foods contain no cholesterol, but it's found in abundance in animal foods, especially egg yolks, red meat, and organ meats. Shellfish contain a relatively large amount of cholesterol, as do dairy products like whole milk, ice cream, butter, and cream cheese.

Cholesterol combines with two different types of lipoproteins that transport it in the body. LDL, or low-density lipoprotein, is bad, or "lousy," cholesterol. It consists of 75 percent cholesterol and comprises the majority of circulating cholesterol. It's important to have some LDL in your system, as it's necessary for cholesterol delivery. However, too much LDL causes cholesterol build-up in the arteries. The oxidizing of LDL can help lead to the development of arteriosclerosis. Since your risk for developing heart disease increases in your menopausal years, be sure to get plenty of antioxidants, such as vitamin A, vitamin C, selenium, reduced glutathione, and alpha lipoic acid, to help keep LDL from oxidizing and causing heart and blood-vessel disease.

High-density lipoprotein, commonly called "good" cholesterol, contains more protein than cholesterol and comprises only about 20 percent to 30 percent of the total cholesterol in the blood. Unlike LDL, HDL has a positive impact, as it removes cholesterol from the artery walls and takes it to the liver, where it is incorporated into bile and removed through the intestinal tract.

Dietary fat and cholesterol are listed separately on food nutrition labels making it easy to know how much of each you're consuming when you rely on pre-packaged products. But many people mistakenly assume that food labeled as "no cholesterol" is also fat-free. Mayonnaise, for example, doesn't have much cholesterol, because it's made from vegetable oil, but it's almost entirely fat. "No cholesterol" doesn't necessarily mean "low calorie" either. Sugar is often added to low-fat/low-cholesterol products to make up for the satisfaction factor that these products often lack.

There is no set standard for optimal fat intake. Most health professionals recommend keeping fat intake at about 30 percent of your total calories, with only 10 percent or less of the fat you eat coming from saturated sources. The American Heart Association recommends consuming no more than 300 mg a day of cholesterol.

It is interesting to note that the human brain in almost 70% cholesterol by weight and

---

The amount of cholesterol in the body is measured through a blood test called a serum lipid profile. The results of that test are represented in several ways:

- **Total cholesterol,** which, as the term suggests, is a measurement of both types of cholesterol. For adults, anything less than 200 mg/dL is considered desirable. Levels in the 200 to 239 mg/dL range are considered borderline high risk. Anything over 240 mg/dL is considered high risk. (These figures and the ones that follow are recommended by the American Heart Association.)

- **HDL cholesterol** (the good stuff). In men and women, the average is 50 to 60 mg/dL. The higher the number, the better. Anything less than 40 mg/dL is considered too low.

- **LDL cholesterol** (the bad stuff). In adults, this number should be from less than 100 mg/dL to 129 mg/dL, with less than 100 mg/dL being optimal.

- **VLDL** (very-low-density lipoprotein) can be even more damaging than LDL to vessel walls. It should be less than 30 and can be calculated (if not revealed in your lipid panel) by taking the total-cholesterol figure and subtracting the HDL and LDL from it. What is left is VLDL.

- **Cholesterol ratio.** This is total cholesterol divided by HDL. It's desirable to keep the ratio below 5:1. The optimum ratio is 3.5.

- **Triglycerides,** which are also measured in a serum lipid test. For these, levels less than 150 mg/dL are considered normal, 150-199 mg/dL is borderline high, 200-499 mg/dL is high, and 500 mg/dL or higher is considered extremely high-risk.

requires significant amounts of essential omega-3 and omega-6 fatty acids as neuro-transmitters. Alzheimer's disease was rarely seen before the early 1950s and has become an epidemic in the last 15 years. This may be due, in part, to the extensive use of fluoridating antidepressants, such as Prozac and Paxil, in combination with cholesterol-lowering drugs and excessive dietary-cholesterol restrictions, as well as to a lack of adequate antioxidant protection in diet and supplementation. Many individuals taking cholesterol-lowering drugs report impaired cognition as a side effect.

The Carb Connection

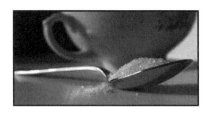

Carbohydrates are the body's primary readily available fuel source. They fall into two categories: simple sugars, which include sweet things like table sugar, honey, maple syrup, fruit sugars, and the like, and complex carbohydrates, which come from plant sources and include grains, vegetables, legumes, beans, and seeds. What differentiates simple carbohydrates from their more complex relatives is their chemical composition. Simple sugars, as the name implies, are relatively simple compounds. When several simple sugars link up, they become a complex carbohydrate.

All carbohydrates, regardless of whether they're simple or complex, are great energy sources, as the body easily digests and breaks them down into glucose—the body's main energy source, which is stored in muscles or the liver. The body can only store a limited amount of carbohydrates, however, so it's important to replace them on a regular basis.

What's the optimal intake level for carbohydrates? This is becoming almost as controversial as fat and protein levels are. Past recommendations ranged anywhere from 45 percent to 75 percent of total daily calories, depending on activity levels and overall health goals. However, high carbohydrate consumption, and especially high consumption of simple carbohydrates, has been shown to be bad for the body, contributing to chronically elevated blood-glucose levels, abnormal insulin levels, high cholesterol levels, metabolic disorders, and some forms of cancer.

These are all serious health concerns, but the effect of carbs on blood-sugar levels, insulin levels, and cholesterol levels are of particular importance for menopausal women, as they are also related to hormone levels.

For the best nutritional benefits, be sure to select your carbohydrates from every food group that contains them—grains, fruits, vegetables, and dairy products.

The average American consumes an average of 135 pounds of refined sugar annually, which equates to a hefty 600 calories a day. This is up substantially from the turn of the 20th century, when the annual per-person consumption of sugar was 65 pounds. According to a study by the USDA, people who eat large amounts of added sugars get less calcium, fiber, folate, vitamins A, C, and E, zinc, magnesium, iron, and other nutrients than people whose diets contain less added sugar.

Simple Sugar Blues

Simple sugars, which are found naturally in certain foods and are added to many processed foods, are a great energy source. Of all the carbohydrates, they get absorbed the fastest. However, the energy burst they provide is temporary. What's more, following a diet high in simple sugars can lead to many health problems, including periodontal disease, hypoglycemia, and diabetes. It can also weaken your immune system.

Simple sugars have almost no redeeming nutritional value, as they are little more than empty calories. This isn't to say that you should avoid all foods that contain them. It is, however a good idea to avoid those that contain refined or processed sugars and to limit your intake of foods that contain naturally occurring simple sugars, such as fruit and fruit juice.

Watching for Hidden Sugars

Even if you stay away from sweets or read food labels carefully, you still can be consuming a large amount of refined sugar without knowing it. Nutritional labels do tally the grams of sugar and grams of total carbohydrates that occur naturally in a product, but they don't have to list any sugars that might be added separately. Because of this, a food product that naturally contains sugar can also contain other types of sugar, such as honey, carob, corn syrup, and fructose, plus a host of other sweetening products. While all the above will be included as part of the total grams of sugar and carbohydrates listed on the label, you won't know how much has come from the sugar, the honey, or the corn syrup, for example.

Even foods that appear to be healthy when you look at the nutrition labels might not seem as great when you scan the actual ingredient lists. If added sugars do appear on such a list, there is, unfortunately, currently no way to know exactly how much has been added. Your only clue is ingredient order, as they're sorted by amount. If sugars are fairly high on the list, they also factor heavily in the food product.

If you want to know if a food has added sugars, look over the ingredient list for the following products:

▸ Sucrose: This is usually processed, granulated white sugar. Other sweeteners that contain sucrose include turbinado sugar, brown sugar, maple syrup, and molasses.

▸ Corn syrup: This is most popular

form of refined fructose. It's sweeter and cheaper than refined sucrose, which makes it a favorite of food manufacturers.

▸ Glucose (or dextrose): Found in fruit, honey, carob, and corn, it can also be refined.

▸ Sugar alcohols (or polyols): These are metabolized more slowly than sucrose and are often recommended for those following diabetic or low-carb diets. They're not completely absorbed by the intestine and can have a laxative effect if too much is eaten. There are a number of different sugar alcohols, including mannitol, sorbitol, maltitol, and xylitol, all of which also occur naturally in fruits.

Other sweeteners that might appear on ingredient lists include fructose, brown sugar, honey, molasses, fruit-juice concentrate, maltose, maltodextrin, lactose, and galactose.

There have been calls for nutrition labels to contain more detailed information on sugars, including a declaration of added sugars in grams per serving and a corresponding daily value, and this information might be added in the future. For now, however, the only way you can tell if a product has added sugars is by reading the ingredient list.

While no sweetener can be considered a nutritional knockout, some are better choices than others when it comes to things like how they affect blood-sugar levels. Some also offer minerals and vitamins.

- Barley malt: This is a dark, sticky sweetener that contains trace amounts of eight vitamins and several minerals. With its strong flavor, it doesn't appeal to everyone but goes well in hearty dishes. Its main ingredient is maltose, and it enters the bloodstream slowly.

- Date sugar: This kind is derived from ground-up, dehydrated dates. Since dates are rich in fiber as well as a wide range of vitamins and minerals, date sugar contains some as well. It works best in baking, when it can be exchanged measure for measure for sugar.

- Fruit-juice concentrates: These fructose-based products are made from the juices of various fruits that are reduced by about one-quarter through slow cooking. They're often used to sweeten and intensify the fla-

vor of juice-concentrate blends. White grape juice is a common fruit-juice concentrate. Be sure to choose those that haven't been stripped of their nutritional value during processing.

- Fructose: Also known as levulose, this simple sugar is derived from fruit sugar and closely resembles granulated white sugar. It's highly concentrated, so you can use less of it to get the same level of sweetness as you get from table sugar. It is believed that fructose doesn't have the same negative effects on blood-sugar levels that sucrose does.

- FruitSource: Made from a mixture of fruit and grains, this product contains both simple and complex carbohydrates as well as small amounts of proteins, fats, vitamins, and minerals. It replaces both sugar and fat in baking and can also be used in beverages and cooking.

- Granular fruit sweeteners: These products are derived from white-grape juice and grain sweeteners that are dehydrated and ground into granules.

- Honey: There are definitely two sides to the story on this sweetener. It can rot teeth faster than sucrose (which it contains), and it can cause fluctuations in blood-sugar levels just as sucrose does. However, it also contains fructose, and the more fructose it contains, the less it affects blood-sugar levels. If you can, use only raw, unfiltered honey, which is minimally processed and contains all of its natural enzymes, proteins, vitamins, and minerals. Unfiltered honey also contains small amounts of bee pollen, which some studies suggest can help control allergies and hay-fever symptoms.

▸ Maltose: Maltose is derived from sprouted grains and cooked rice, which are mixed with natural enzymes and heated until the starch they contain turns into sugar. Maltose is about one-third as sweet as sucrose. Barley malt and brown-rice syrup are two natural sweeteners that contain maltose.

▸ Maple syrup: The boiled-down sap of maple trees contains twice as much calcium as milk does. Some syrups also contain traces of formaldehyde, so choose organic maple syrup if possible.

▸ Rice syrup: Mild in flavor, this traditional Asian sweetener contains trace

amounts of B vitamins and minerals. It can be used instead of honey in cooking and baking and to sweeten beverages and cereals.

▸ Sorghum syrup: This old-fashioned sweetener comes from the sorghum cane.

▸ Stevia: Derived from a South American shrub, this herb can give foods a sweet taste. It is sold as a dietary supplement rather than a sweetener, as the FDA considers it an unapproved food additive. Stevia has no dietary carbohydrate value because it does not get absorbed.

▸ Sucanat: This product is made from evaporated sugar-cane juice and contains vitamins, minerals, and trace elements. It has a distinct flavor, similar to that of molasses, which can take some getting used to. It can be used as an equal replacement for sugar in baking and cooking and in hot or cold drinks.

▸ Unsulfured blackstrap molasses: There are several different types of molasses; unsulfered blackstrap molasses is what's left from cane syrup after the sugar crystals are removed from it. It contains high levels of three important minerals—calcium, iron, and potassium.

What About Sugar Substitutes?

Sugar substitutes are at least 30 times sweeter than sucrose. Saccharin, aspartame (marketed as Nutrasweet, Equal, and Spoonful), acesulfame potassium (marketed as Sunette), and sucralose with dextrose and maltodextrin (marketed as Splenda) have all been approved by the FDA for consumer use. In reviewing these, the best-tasting, safest product, free of dietary sugars seems to be Splenda.

Although there are no set dietary guidelines for added sugars (yet), the U.S. Department of Agriculture suggests limiting added sugars to 40 grams (10 teaspoons) for a 2,000-calorie diet.

The jury is still out over the benefits of using artificial sweeteners. Some studies suggest that people who use them to shave calories end up getting those calories somewhere else, or that they actually increase hunger. Some people also report undesirable side effects from a number of artificial sweeteners.

Weight gain is often an issue as a woman enters menopause. It's important when entering menopause to balance the amounts of protein, carbohydrates, and fat you are getting with regular aerobic and weight-bearing exercise. Properly balancing one's diet and exercise is an essential part of a complete treatment plan for optimal hormonal health.

Complex Carbs

Complex carbohydrates are foods that contain linked simple sugars and are structurally more complex. The body also turns complex carbohydrates into glucose, but it does it more slowly due to the more complex chemical structure of these foods.

Choosing whole grains and minimally processed carbohydrates over highly processed/sugary carbs helps regulate blood-sugar levels. However, complex carbs that have a low glycemic index (GI) are better choices than others.

The Glycemic Index and Blood-sugar Levels

The glycemic index is a tool that measures how foods affect blood-glucose levels. As a benchmark you can look at pure glucose, which is at 100 on the index. Foods that break down the fastest and affect blood-glucose levels the fastest are at the high end of the scale (closer to 100). Some are so high on the GI index, like dextrose at 138, that they even score higher than 100. GI ratings of greater than 70 are considered high; 55 or less is considered low.

The following are examples of foods at the high end of the glycemic chart:

Table 8: Glycemic-index Rating

Food	Glycemic-index Rating
dates	103
sticky rice	98
baked potato	93
corn flakes	92
rice crackers	91
wild rice	87
pretzels	83
bagel	72
popcorn	72
watermelon	72
corn, fresh	60

Foods with lower, more favorable, glycemic indexes include the following:

Table 9: Glycemic-index Rating

Food	Glycemic-index Rating
brown rice	55
oatmeal	55
kidney beans, canned	52
butter	47
all bran w/fiber	38
apple	38
pear, fresh	38
tomato juice	38
whole milk	31
apricots, dried	30
lentils	29
prunes	29
cherries	22
grapefruit	25
peanut butter	14
yogurt, artificially sweetened	14
broccoli	10
lettuce	10
mushrooms	10
hummus	6

The glycemic index has received some undeserved bad press because people have misunderstood how to use it. The chemistry behind the concept is complex and isn't that important to understand, but it is important to know that foods on the high end of the glycemic level, such as white sugar, processed grain products, and other carbohydrates that are high in simple sugars, send blood-glucose levels soaring, which means that the body has to release more insulin to bring them down.

If you rely too heavily on foods with high GI levels your body has to keep manufacturing more insulin to combat the spikes in blood sugar that they cause. Researchers now believe that increased insulin levels encourage the body to store calories as fat. They also cause cells to become insulin-resistant. The result: obesity and diabetes, which, I don't have to tell you, are both reaching epidemic proportions in our modern society.

Eating slow-release, low-GI food, such as whole-wheat pasta, stone-ground whole-wheat bread, high-fiber fruits and vegetables, and foods that contain fat and protein puts lower and slower doses of glucose into your bloodstream and reduces the workload on your pancreas. It also keeps you from experiencing wild swings in your blood-sugar levels, which can cause headaches, "brain fog", and irritability among other symptoms.

Monosaccharides—the Simplest of Sugars

In addition to the simple sugars that we are familiar with, such as glucose and fructose, there are simpler sugars known as monosaccharides. These monosaccharides are our building blocks and cell-to-cell communicators. The monosaccharides combine in a stacked fashion to form saccharide chains, complex proteins, and lipids, which in turn form glycoproteins and glycolipids. These complexes orchestrate the nutrient exchange into and out of the cells, aid in cell-to-cell communication, and play a crucial role in cell repair and wound healing all while maintaining the highways between our cells called gap junctions.

As our lives become more challenged with a range of hormonal imbalances and nutrient deficiencies, we become unable to biosynthesize some of these monosaccharides in the correct amounts. Glyconutrients have been developed as supplements to provide these monosaccharides in adequate amounts. They can significantly improve hormone-receptor binding and cell uptake. See the resource section at the back of this book for information on how to purchase quality glyconutrients.

Fiber Facts

Another benefit of eating more complex carbohydrates is that you naturally end up taking in more fiber. Studies have linked high-fiber intake with lower occurrences of some serious medical problems, including heart disease, diabetes, obesity, intestinal disorders, hypertension, and several types of cancer, including colorectal cancer, prostate cancer, and breast cancer.

> The fibrous part of carbohydrates contains the greatest concentrations of vitamins, minerals, and disease-fighting antioxidants.

Fiber is the exclusive substance of the plant world. It makes up the flesh of all non-animal foods as well as their leaves, stems, roots, seeds, and coverings. There are various types of fiber in plants. Cellulose, the most abundant organic molecule on Earth, is primarily contained inside of plant-cell walls. Another common fiber, called mucilage is found within plant cells.

The human body can't digest fiber, so what we take in passes right through. As it does, however, it helps to promote good health. Soluble fiber, found in oats, beans, peas, seeds, certain fruits and vegetables, and psyllium, clings to cholesterol and removes it from the body. Insoluble fiber, which passes through the system largely intact, increases stool bulk and speeds up its transit through the intestinal tract, which helps prevent constipation and irritable bowel syndrome and also helps reduce the risk of one's developing hemorrhoids and diverticulosis. It's found in whole grains, wheat bran, nuts, seeds, and the stalks and peels of fruits and vegetables.

Other fiber benefits include:

▸ It slows down the rate at which carbohydrates are digested, resulting in slower and steadier glucose release.

▸ It contains micronutrients, particularly magnesium, which may help prevent diabetes.

▸ It expands in your stomach when you eat it, helping you feel full longer.

▸ It binds cholesterol and increases its excretion through the bowel.

The typical Western diet, with its emphasis on fiber-free animal foods and processed foods that often have most of their natural fiber removed, is extremely low in fiber. In fact, the average American only eats roughly 12 to 15 grams of fiber a day; that's far below the 20 to 35 grams recommended in the FDA's dietary guidelines. In comparison, people living in Africa and India take in between 40 and 150 grams of fiber a day.

The current recommendation is for 20 to 35 grams of fiber a day. However, some experts recommend levels as high as 60 grams a day. It's better to get your fiber from food than from over-the-counter supplements. Doing so will also provide other important

The Top 10 Food Sources of Fiber

Food	Fiber (grams)
❶ beans (legumes), cooked, 1 cup	12
❷ peas, green, cooked, 1 cup	9
❸ raspberries, 1 cup	8
❹ bulgur, cooked, 1 cup	8
❺ rye wafers, 3 crackers	7
❻ wheat bran, 1/4 cup	6
❼ pasta, whole-wheat, cooked, 1 cup	6
❽ oat bran, cooked, 1 cup	6
❾ squash, acorn, 4 oz.	5
❿ potato, baked with skin, 1 medium	5

Table 8: The Top 10 Food Sources of Fiber

nutrients. However, fiber supplements can be used to reach these levels. Good ones have a 2:1 or 3:1 ratio of soluble to insoluble fiber for maximum health benefits. Supplements containing psyllium, derived from a plant native to India and Iran, are especially high in fiber.

It's best to increase fiber intake slowly. Even in small amounts, eating more fiber can cause gas and intestinal cramps until your system adjusts to it. These are common but temporary side effects that typically disappear in a few weeks. If they bother you excessively, simply cut back on how much you are eating. There are also dietary supplements you can try—Beano is one—to help ease your way into a fiber-full life. Be sure that your fluid intake is what it should be as well. Fiber needs water to expand in the gut and move on through.

Another great source of fiber is organic flaxseeds, freshly ground into a powder and added to a daily smoothie. Flaxseeds are an excellent source of soluble and insoluble fiber, and their mucilage functions as a stool softener, enhancing the fiber's effect. The mucilage also soothes the colon and promotes the growth of friendly probiotic bacteria, making flaxseeds a perfect choice for increasing fiber in the diet. Since the seeds' outer shells are indigestible, you must eat the seeds ground up to obtain the valuable EFAs and lignans contained within the kernels. However, flaxseed meal is extremely unstable and will rapidly deteriorate within 24 hours of milling. Once rancid, a food that was bursting with health-protective attributes becomes a source of damaging free radicals. I recommend purchasing organic flaxseeds whole and grinding them fresh daily.

The proper ratio of protein, carbohydrates, fats and fiber in your diet will depend on the type of diet you are following. People on a very-high-protein diet (diabetics, for example) need to supplement with plenty of fiber as well as a drinking plenty of water. High protein dieters should also be neutralizing acidity with coral calcium or some other alkalinizing calcium source.

The Best Menopause Diet

While recommending a specific eating plan is beyond the scope of this book, this chapter should give you enough basic knowledge to start developing one of your own. You'll also find some resources for doing so in the resource section at the back of this book.

There are many different approaches to eating for good health, and not a great deal of agreement on which one is best. Based on research, however, it's been found that women in their menopausal years do best when they follow diets that are lower in carbohydrates than what has been previously recommended.

Many health professionals feel that an ideal balance of protein/carbs/fats for menopausal women is 30%:40%:30%. This ratio provides a good balance of fats and proteins to stabilize blood sugar and keep your insulin levels low. If your typical daily intake of calories is 1,800—the high end of the scale for recommended calorie intake for women—your protein intake should be 30 percent of this—540 calories, or 135 grams of protein. If, on the other hand, you're on the low end at 1,200 calories, your protein intake should be 360 calories, or 90 grams of protein.

This level of protein intake really doesn't equate to a lot of food, especially if you're eating animal protein. If you split it up over three meals and two snacks (also recommended for maintaining consistent blood-sugar levels), it would be about a 3-oz. serving of animal protein for each of at your main meals and 1 to 2-oz. servings for snacks. If you substitute some plant proteins (legumes, nuts, and seeds) for animal proteins you'll be able to eat more.

Other recommendations for eating right for menopause and beyond include the following:

▸ Eat a wide variety of foods from all food groups.

▸ Choose low-fat protein sources that come from producers who don't use hormones on their animals.

▸ Substitute plant proteins for animal proteins on a regular basis. Soy products have some of the highest protein levels of all plant proteins and are a source of health-enhancing phytoestrogens.

▸ Avoid foods that contain simple sugars (candy, baked goods, and the like). Read labels carefully for added sugars that aren't declared on nutrition labeling.

▸ Choose healthy fats over unhealthy ones. Avoid products with transfatty acids whenever possible.

▸ Choose foods that are high in fiber.

▸ Choose whole foods over processed ones whenever possible.

▸ Strive for a minimum of three ½-cup servings of vegetables daily. Limit fruit to two ½-cup servings.

▸ Choose whole-grain products over processed ones.

▸ Try to eat foods that are high in calcium. Many people, especially as they get older, don't like the taste of dairy foods, or find them hard to digest. If you're in the latter group, try lactose-reduced products. If , however, you simply don't like the taste of dairy products, you'll need to take calcium supplements, which I'll discuss in Chapter 8.

▸ Drink plenty of water, minimally 16 ounces upon rising, 16 ounces one hour before bedtime, and 32 ounces throughout the day. Drink more if you weigh over 150 lbs.

▸ Supplement with essential fatty acids, vitamins, minerals, trace minerals, antioxidants, and glyconutrients.

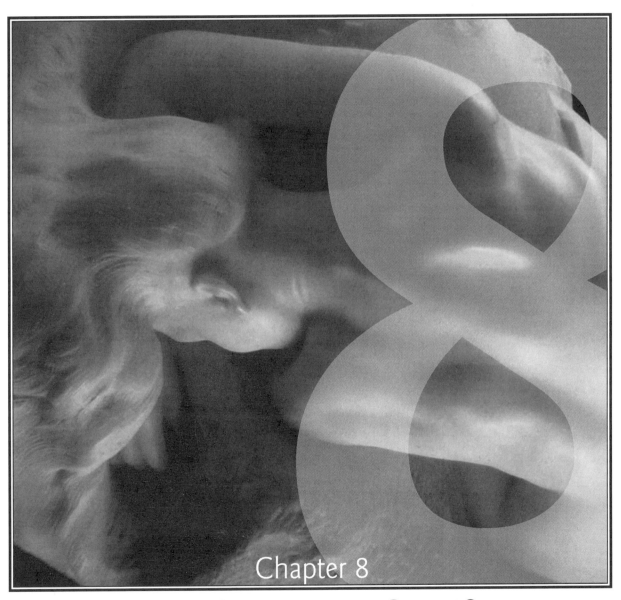

Chapter 8

Supplementing for Life

Chapter 8
Supplementing for Life

Vitamins and minerals (or micronutrients) are the substances the body needs to put macronutrients to work. They don't contain energy of their own, but they are essential for releasing energy from food. They also play a key role in tissue growth, healing, and repair.

The role that these nutrients play in good health has been known for some time, but only in the last 20 years or so has vitamin and mineral supplementation really taken off. Not only do we know a great deal more about how they work and their importance in maintaining good health, but there is a greater need today for taking supplemental vitamins and minerals than ever before. Experts used to believe that people could get all the necessary vitamins and minerals if they followed a balanced diet and ate the right amount of food. The problem is, however, that most people don't do either of those things.

To make things even more tricky research has also shown that many foods today don't contain the same levels of vitamins and minerals that they once did. For this reason, it is difficult to impossible to eat enough of some of these foods to meet the recommended daily requirements for certain vitamins—not to mention to reach the higher levels of some micronutrients needed for protection against certain chronic and degenerative illnesses.

There are 13 vitamins and about 22 minerals that the body needs to keep operating as it should. A reference system called the dietary reference intakes, or DRIs, determines how much of these substances are necessary for basic good health.

A two-year study of Americans' eating habits conducted by the U.S. Department of Agriculture found that more than 80 percent of women and more than 70 percent of men consumed less than two-thirds of the RDA for one or more micronutrients. Fewer than half the participants met the RDAs for vitamins A, B_6, and E or for calcium, magnesium, and zinc.

About Daily Values

DRIs are the newest take on the recommended dietary allowances (RDAs) published more than 60 years ago by the Food and Nutrition Board of the National Academy of Sciences. The earlier guidelines recommended nutrient-intake levels that experts believed would meet the nutritional needs for most healthy people, and were based on research that was available at the time. The new guidelines take into account the different nutritional needs of various populations, and provide several values for each nutrient instead of just one. The new values are also based more on the philosophy of preventing chronic diseases than that of preventing nutritional deficiencies.

The DRI system offers guidelines for both recommended and maximum intake amounts. It uses the following reference values:

▸ Recommended dietary allowance (RDA): This is the intake level that meets the nutrient needs of almost all healthy individuals in specific age and gender groups.

▸ Estimated average requirement (EAR):

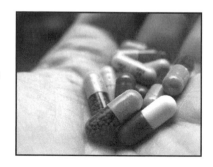

This is the nutrient level determined to meet the needs of 50 percent of individuals in a specific group. It is based on strong research evidence and is used to determine a nutrient's RDA.

▸ Adequate intake (AI): Adequate intake is set when there aren't enough data to establish an RDA. These figures are less precise than RDAs but will still meet or exceed the nutrient needs for almost all healthy people.

▸ Tolerable upper limit (UL): This is the highest vitamin or mineral level that can be safely taken without risking adverse health effects. It can't be set for all nutrients, due to a lack of scientific information for some of them.

I have included charts here that show the current RDA (also called RDI, for Reference daily intake, or DRV, for daily reference value, or just DV, for daily value) for adults and the new DRI levels for women.

Vitamin-intake Levels

Vitamin	Current RDA	New DRI
A	5,000 IU	900 mcg
C	60 mg	90 mg
D	400 IU	15 mcg
E	30 IU	15 mg
K	80 mcg	120 mcg
thiamin	1.5 mg	1.2 mg
riboflavin	1.7 mg	1.3 mg
niacin	20 mg	16 mg
vitamin B_6	2 mg	1.7 mg
folate	400 mcg	400 mcg from food, 200 mcg synthetic
vitamin B_{12}	6 mcg	2.4 mcg
biotin	300 mcg	30 mcg
pantothenic	10 mg	5 mg
choline	not established	550 mg

Table 9: Vitamin-intake Levels

(Source: Institute of Medicine, National Academies of Science, Council for Responsible Nutrition)

Mineral Consumption Levels

Mineral	Current RDA	New DRI
calcium	1,000 mg	1,300 mg
iron	18 mg	18 mg for pre-menopause, 8 mg/day for post-menopause
phosphorus	1,000 mg	700 mg
iodine	150 mcg	150 mcg
magnesium	400 mg	320 mg
zinc	15 mg	8 mg
selenium	70 mcg	55 mcg
copper	2 mg	900 mcg
manganese	2 mg	1.8 mg
chromium	120 mcg	25 mcg
molybdenum	75 mcg	45 mcg

Table 10: Mineral Consumption Levels

(Source: Institute of Medicine, National Academies of Science, Council for Responsible Nutrition)

The Food and Nutrition Board of the National Academy of Sciences, or FNB, also set new guidelines for mineral consumption. See Table 10 for details.

These figures represent only the nutrient levels that have been established to meet *basic* health needs. Current research has shown that higher intakes of certain vitamins and minerals are necessary to prevent many chronic and

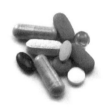

degenerative diseases.

For perimenopausal and menopausal women, there are some vitamins and minerals that are particularly important to know about—which I'll discuss later in this chapter.

Vital Vitamins

The human body needs 13 vitamins for growth, protection, and energy regulation. It can't make these vitamins, or at least can't make enough of them, so they must be obtained from outside sources. Vitamins come in two forms:

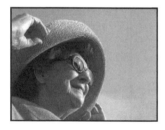

▸ Fat-soluble ones (A, E, D, K): These vitamins are stored in the body's fat and liver, where they stay until they're needed. Taking too much of them can be dangerous.

▸ Water-soluble ones (B_1, B_2, B_6, B_{12}, niacin, pantothenic acid, folic acid, biotin, and vitamin C): These vitamins are excreted in the urine if you take too much of them.

The majority of the vitamins are obtained from food. However, not all food is created equal when it comes to vitamin content. Vitamin levels can differ significantly depending on how food is grown and where it is grown. How food is shipped, stored, bought, and cooked can also affect nutrient levels.

Necessary Minerals

For good health, the body also requires at least 50 different mineral substances in varying amounts. The key players are the macrominerals, which are seven important substances that your body needs in amounts ranging from a fraction of a gram to several grams. Also important, but in smaller amounts, are trace minerals or microminerals, which are measured in milligrams and micrograms. There are also microtrace, ultratrace, are rare earth minerals, which are measured in parts per million (ppm).

Minerals are as important as vitamins and in some respects even more so, as they enable vitamins to do their work. Unlike vitamins,

Vitamins

Vitamin	Functions	Dietary sources
A	vision, mucous- membrane formation, liver, bone, and tooth growth, growth and repair of one's body structure, healthy skin, immune function	dark-green and deep-orange vegetables, beef liver, fortified milk, cheese, egg yolks
D (calciferol)	bone growth and health, increased calcium and phosphorous absorption	cod liver oil, eggs, dairy products, fortified milk, margarine
E (tocopherol)	antioxidant qualities, prevents cell damage, anticoagulant qualities	seeds, nuts, green leafy vegetables, margarine, shortenings, wheat germ
K (phylloquinone)	blood clotting, glycogen formation	liver, green leafy vegetables, small amounts in cereals, fruit, meats, milk, yogurt
B_1 (thiamine)	energy metabolism, nervous-system function, muscle tone, heart function	pork, organ meats, whole grains, nuts, legumes, milk, fruits, vegetables, dried yeast
B_2 (riboflavin)	Energy metabolism, maintenance of eye tissue, cellular respiration	meats, eggs, milk products, whole-grain and enriched cereal products, wheat germ, green leafy vegetables
B_3 (niacin)	energy metabolism, skin, nervous system and digestive tract health, formation of red blood cells	milk, eggs, meat, poultry, legumes, peanuts, fish, mushrooms, greens, dried yeast, liver
B_6 (pyridoxine)	energy metabolism, red-blood-cell production, nervous-system function, healthy skin	meats, fish, poultry, vegetables, whole grains, cereals, seeds, dried yeast, organ meats, liver, peanuts, walnuts, dried beans, avocados
Pantothenic acid	supports adrenal glands, support of healthy skin and nerves, metabolization of carbohydrates and fats into energy, necessary for making fatty acids, cholesterol, and steroids	meat, fish, poultry, milk products, legumes, whole grains, liver, yeast
Folate (folic acid, folacin)	DNA and RNA synthesis, regulation of growth, breakdown of proteins, maturation of red blood cells, protection against neurological defects in newborns	legumes, green vegetables, whole wheat products, meats, eggs, milk product, liver, dried yeast, wheat germ, sweet potatoes
B_{12} (cobalamin)	cell synthesis, nerve function, metabolism of carbohydrates, proteins and fat, formation of red blood cells	muscle meats, fish, eggs, dairy products
Biotin	fatty acid and carbohydrate metabolism	legumes, vegetables, meats, liver, egg yolk, cauliflower, yeast, nuts
Vitamin C	collagen formation, amino acid metabolism, enhanced iron absorption, antioxidant qualities, bone and connective tissue growth, wound repair	citrus fruits, tomatoes, green peppers, salad greens, potatoes, cabbage, broccoli

Table 11: Vital Vitamins

minerals can't be destroyed by food handling, processing, cooking, or storage.

Our soil has been depleted of trace minerals throughout the 20th century as a result of farming techniques that call for refertilizing the soil with only three minerals; nitrogen, phosphorus, and potassium (N-P-K). While it's true that these three minerals are the only ones necessary to maximize crop yield, your body needs all the essential minerals to function optimally. To use an analogy, think of the essential nutrients and minerals as tools in the body's toolbox for repair, rejuvenation, and longevity. Without all the necessary tools, certain problems literally cannot be fixed and parts of our body can't work properly anymore. To make matters worse, a number of events of the 20th century have added to demineralizing us as a culture. They include the following:

1. The damming of our rivers, reducing irrigation with mineralized mountain and river water.

2. The transition from wood stoves to electric and propane stoves in the early 1940s. According to the epidemiological and anthropological research of Joel Wallach, B.S. (agriculture), D.V.M., N.D. this tran-

sition abruptly stopped the recycling of wood ash into our gardens to aid in mineralizing our crops. This natural life cycle of wood ash remineralization of soil had occurred without interruption throughout all prior cultures worldwide.

3. The dramatic drop in home gardening's being replaced with commercial farming.

The reduction, or absence, of many of the more than 50 essential minerals has led to a broad-based mineral depletion in our diet. Soils fertilized only with N-P-K are gradually depleted of the other essential minerals. After a 5 to 15 year period, there are no significant minerals in the soil, the plants that grow in it, and the animals that graze on the depleted fields. N-P-K has been used as exclusive fertilizing in commercial farming since the early 1900s. Our soils have been demineralized for the last 75 to 100 years, and, as a result we as an entire culture have been demineralized!

Plants can manufacture vitamins through photosynthesis. However, plants can't make minerals. The plant relies on the soil it grows in to have adequate mineral content to be taken up by the plant and made available to us for consumption in a highly absorbable form. Humans are meant to take in minerals through plants and animals that have eaten plants rich in minerals, trace minerals, and rare earth minerals from naturally mineral-rich soils. Soil-based sources of minerals are much more bioavailable—up to 98%—as compared with minerals derived from limestone, oyster shells, or other rocklike sources that hover around a 2% to 10% absorption rate. Amino-acid chelates can increase absorption up to 40%.

Joel Wallach, D.V.M, N.D. and a classmate of mine during medical-school training at the National College of Naturopathic Medicine (1979-1983) has written several wonderful books outlining the essential value of electrolytes, macrominerals, trace minerals, and rare earth minerals in human physiology. I refer you to his books titled <u>Dead Doctors Don't Lie</u> , <u>Rare Earth's Forbidden Cures</u>, and <u>Hell's Kitchen</u> for a much more complete discussion of this very important subject. See the resource section at the back of this book for information on quality plant-derived colloidal trace minerals and Dr. Wallach's books.

About Antioxidants

Antioxidants are the big news these days. This special group of vitamins, minerals, and vitaminlike phyto nutrients works to protect the body from free radicals that impair the human body and cause it to age.

Free radicals are caused, interestingly enough, by the oxygen we use to make energy. The byproducts left over from this process, called free radicals (single oxygen molecules), differ from other atoms in the body in that they either are short an electron or have one too many. To regain their balance, they steal electrons from other atoms. When searching for that extra electron, they damage whatever is around them, including cell DNA, membranes and walls, blood vessels, and proteins and fats.

Free radicals are always present in the body. Antioxidants work to keep them in check. However, free radicals can duplicate and make more free radicals, thanks to a phenomenon called oxidative stress, which develops when the free radicals in the body outnumber antioxidants.

Major Minerals and Their Functions

The following chart discusses the more major minerals and their known functions.

Major Macrominerals and Electrolytes	Function	Dietary Sources
Calcium	Bone and tooth formation. Blood clotting. Nerve transmission. Smooth-muscle contraction.	Milk, cheese, dark-green vegetables, dried legumes.
Chlorin	An important component of extracellular fluids. Electrolyte balance.	Salt-containing foods and some vegetables and fruits.
Magnesium	Activates enzymes involved in protein synthesis. Aids in muscle relaxation. Helps metabolize carbohydrates and proteins. Involved in bone and tooth formation. Regulates body temperature and energy.	Legumes, nuts, artichokes, avocados, corn, halibut, mackerel, peas, tofu, cocoa, leafy green vegetables, whole-grain cereals and breads, soybeans.
Phosphorus	Bone and tooth formation. Essential for energy production. Helps maintain acid-base balance.	Milk, cheese, yogurt, meat, poultry, grains, fish, legumes, and nuts.
Potassium	Fluid-based nerve transmission. Carbohydrate metabolism. Protein synthesis.	Leafy vegetables, cantaloupes, lima beans, potatoes, bananas, milk, meats, coffee, tea, prunes, raisins, oranges, potassium chloride in salt replacements.
Sodium	Helps maintain acid-base balance, aids nerve function.	Common salt, beef, pork, sardines, green olives, sauerkraut, cheese.
Sulfur	Helps maintain acid-base balance. Aids with liver function. Appears to stabilize protein molecules in the body (especially in the hair, nails, and skin).	Thiamine, insulin, methionine, and cysteine. Also used as a food preservative.

Table 12: Major Minerals and Their Functions

Minor Minerals and Their Functions

There are many minerals listed below such as selenium and boron that are now considered essential and in the past where thought to be toxic and of no essential value.

Minor Minerals	Function	Dietary Sources	Minor Minerals	Function	Dietary Sources
Boron	Brain function. Bone growth, repair, and maintenance. May help increase the levels of certain hormones.	Fruit-based beverages and other products, potatoes, legumes, milk, avocados, peanut butter, and peanuts.	Nickel	Is a cofactor for metalloenzymes. Enhances gastrointestinal absorption of iron and zinc.	Beans, peas, nuts, oatmeal, chocolate.
Chromium	Essential for removal of sugar and fat. Metabolism. Maintaining blood-glucose levels.	Legumes, cereals, organ meats.	Selenium	Protects cells from free-radical damage. Softens fibrous tissues as in uterine fibroids, fibrocystic breasts, and fibromyalgia. Cofactor in the conversion of T4 thyroxin into its active form, T3.	Seafood, meats, milk, eggs, grains.
Copper	Manufacturing red blood cells, nerves, and collagen. Aids iron absorption and transport. and thyroid metabolism. Maintains artery, vein walls and hair pigment.	Meats, drinking water, nuts, shellfish, organ meats, grains, legumes, dark leafy vegetables.	Silicon	Increases collagen in growing bone up to 100%. Aids in hair, skin, bone and fingernail growth.	Whole grains, beets, bell peppers, beans, peas.
Fluoride	May be important in maintaining bone structure	Drinking water, tea, coffee, seafood.	Tin	Induces the enzyme heme oxygenase. Protects against hearing and hair loss.	Canned foods.
Iodine	Formation of thyroid hormones that regulate metabolism.	Seafood, dairy products, vegetables, iodized salt, some drinking water.	Vanadium	Necessary for normal iodine metabolism and thyroid function. Blood-sugar oxidation and transport in fat cells, the liver, and muscles. Stimulates insulin's effect on DNA synthesis. Lowers cholesterol.	Parsley, black pepper, dill, mushrooms, and shellfish.
Iron	Transporting oxygen in the bloodstream. Immune functions. Prevents anemia.	Eggs, lean meats, legumes, whole grains, green leafy vegetables, soybean flour, prune juice, chicken, tuna.	Zinc	Detoxification of alcohol. Boosts the immune system. Helps maintain healthy skin. Assists in protein digestion. Aids in DNA and RNA synthesis. Assists in normal insulin activity and wound healing.	Shellfish, legumes, organ meat, poultry, pork, seeds, meat, wild rice, wheat germ, cashews, yogurt.
Manganese	Important for skin, bones, and menstrual-cycle maintenance. Used for cholesterol, glucose, and fatty-acid metabolism.	Peanuts, pecans, oatmeal, juice, some cereals, dried fruits, tea, pineapple.			
Molybdenum	Is a cofactor of several enzymes involved in protein and iron metabolism.	Legumes, grain products, cereals, leafy vegetables, nuts.			

Table 13: Minor Minerals and Their Functions

Some factors outside the body can also accelerate free-radical growth, including the following:

- pollutants in the water, food, and air
- ultraviolet rays and ionizing radiation from the sun
- high stress levels
- too little or too much exercise
- smoking and secondhand smoke
- poor dietary habits
- chronic constipation

Free radicals have also been shown to be a key contributor to many disorders that were once thought to be simply a part of the aging process, such as cancer, rheumatoid arthritis, Alzheimer's disease, heart attacks, and strokes.

Eating healthily, exercising moderately, and taking antioxidant supplements can protect against free-radical damage. For optimal cell nutrition, it is important to take higher doses of vitamins with antioxidant properties than of the other micronutrients. Doing so will give your body the best defense against degenerative diseases.

There are many different kinds of free radicals, which means that no single antioxidant will wipe them all out. For this reason, it's a good idea to take a variety of antioxidants or a supplement that contains a variety of them.

The following chart lists the main categories of antioxidants and related vitamins and minerals, their best forms, and their recommended daily values, usually beyond the RDA, and ranging to higher therapeutic amounts. With some antioxidants, you'll want, as noted, a mix of the different forms, because your body will use them better.

In my opinion, some of the better, well-researched antioxidant formulas include those used in several American Longevity products, OPCT, Beyond Juice, Beyond Vegetable, and Vitale. See the resource section under Wellness Revolution in the back of the book for details.

Glyconutrients with a fruit and vegetable base with quercetin, grape extract, green tea, and Australian bush plum have been identified as having a very high ORAC (oxygen reactive absorbance capacity) for both water-soluble and fat-soluble free radicals, retaining this ability to gobble up free radicals for over one year after capsulation. See the resource section (Wellness Revolution) in the back of the book for details.

Antioxidant	Form	Amount
Vitamin A	betacarotine	10,000-15,000 IU
	alpha carotene	500-800 mcg
	lutein/zeaxanthin	1-6 mg
	lycopene*	1-3 mg
Vitamin C	calcium	1,000-2,000 mg
	potassium	
	magnesium	
	zinc ascorbates	
Vitamin D	cholecalciferol	400-800 IU
Vitamin E	d-alpha tocopherol	400-800 IU
	d-gamma tocopherol	
	mixed tocotrienol	
Vitamin K	phylloquinone	50-100 mcg
Alpha-lipolic acid	alpha-lipolic acid	50-1000 mg
Vitamin B_1	thiamin HCL	20-100 mg
Vitamin B_2	riboflavin	25-100 mg
Vitamin B_3	niacin and	30-75 mg
	niacinamide	50-2,000 mg
Vitamin B_5	pantothenic acid,	80-200 mg
	as D-calcium	
	pantothenate	
Vitamin B_6	pyridoxine	25-100 mg
Vitamin B_{12}	cyanocobalamin	100-250 mcg
Biotin	in multi vitamins and	300-1,000 mcg
	B-vitamin compex	
Folate	folic acid	800-1,000 mcg
Bilberry		Amounts vary
Broccoli		Amounts vary

Antioxidant	Form	Amount
Bromelain		Amounts vary
Gingko biloba		Amounts vary
Grapeseed Extract		30-90 mg
Green Tea		Amounts vary
Hawthorne		Amounts vary
Quercetin		Amounts vary
Rutin		Amounts vary
Silymarin		Amounts vary
Calcium	calcium citrate,	800-1500 mg
	calcium triphospate	
	calcium hydroxyapatite	
Chromium	polynicotinate	200-400 mcg
	picolinate	
Copper	copper gluconate	1-3 mg
Iodine	potassium iodine	100-200 mcg
Magnesium	magnesium citrate	500-800 mg
	amino acid	
Manganese	manganese gluconate	3-10 mg
Molybdenum	molybdenum citrate	50-100 mcg
Vanadium	vanadyl sulfate	30-100 mcg
Zinc	zinc citrate	20-50 mg
CoQ10		15-30 mg
	with health challenges	100-600 mg
Glutathione		10-20 mg
Choline	Choline Bitartrate	100-200 mg
Inositol		150-250 mg
Olivol	Olive Extract	30 mg

Table 14: Antioxidants

* Take a mixed carotenoid containing all of these substances. The body
  converts what it needs of the alphacarotine and betacarotine to vitamin A
  and uses the other carotenoids as antioxidants.

Important Vitamins and Minerals for Menopause

There is a group of vitamins and minerals that perimenopausal and menopausal women need to be particularly concerned about. Imbalances of these important nutrients can contribute to a number of problems, including bloating, nervousness, irritability, anxiety, and insomnia. They can also contribute to osteoporosis and cardiovascular problems.

It's possible to get adequate levels of most of these vitamins through food and a good multivitamin/multimineral supplement that is formulated as an antioxidant. There are also supplements that are specially formulated for menopause support, many of which contain the necessary levels of these important nutrients. Additional supplementation might be required for several of them, as noted below.

Calcium

As the most abundant mineral in the body, calcium combines with phosphorus to build bones and teeth. Calcium that circulates in the blood enables muscles to contract. It also aids in blood clotting, in transmitting nerve impulses, in regulating acidity and the acid-base balance, and in moving fluids in and out of cells.

Adequate amounts of calcium are needed throughout life to keep bones strong. However, most adults don't get nearly enough of it on a daily basis. There are also a number of factors that can cause calcium to not be absorbed properly, including the following:

▸ too much protein

▸ excessive alcohol consumption

▸ high-fiber foods

▸ large doses of zinc

▸ oxalic acids (contained in some foods)

▸ uric acids

▸ high caffeine consumption

▸ aluminum hydroxide (found in some antacids)

▸ cigarette smoking

▸ non-weight-bearing exercise

▸ low magnesium intake

▸ excess intake of dietary phosphorous (red meat, soft drinks)

Eating three to four servings of dairy products is recommended to make sure you are getting enough calcium. Dark-green, leafy vegetables also contain calcium, but in substantially lower quantities. However, supplementation is often necessary to meet the minimum RDA (1,000 mg) for this important micronutrient and is almost always needed to reach the higher level (1,300 mg) now recommended for women. The minimum amount may need to increase to 1,250 to 1,500 mg, depending on calcium absorption, bone density, and other health problems that may accompany menopause. Not all calcium supplementation is the same. See the resource section at the back of this book for information on the availability of optimal calcium supplementation.

Blood-calcium levels are often erroneously used to measure bone density, but they're actually not a good indication of it. If blood is lacking calcium, the body will pull it from bone. For this reason, high levels of blood calcium don't necessarily equate to adequate bone-calcium stores. In order to determine bone density, a bone-density-analysis special X-ray of your hips and lower back, called a DexaScan, needs to be performed.

Vitamin D

Vitamin D, which the body makes when exposed to the sun, is essential for proper calcium absorption. Unfortunately, the body's ability to synthesize this vitamin declines with age. Decreased exposure to the sun, either through sunscreen use or simply from spending less time outdoors, also diminishes vitamin D levels in the body.

A study by the National Institute on Aging found that postmenopausal women with too little vitamin D in their diets have an increased risk of hip fracture. You can boost Vitamin D by spending more time outdoors or by using a sunscreen that allows more of the sun's rays to penetrate the skin. To ensure adequate levels, however, it's best to supplement with 400 IUs daily.

Magnesium

Magnesium assists calcium absorption and is another important nutrient for bone health. It's also essential for proper muscle and nerve function, energy metabolism, and hormone transmission. Low magnesium levels can cause heart palpitations and migraine headaches. It can also contribute to depression, mood swings, fatigue, blood-sugar imbalances, and PMS symptoms. Taking a supplement that provides 500 to 1,000 mg per day is recommended.

Zinc

Zinc, which assists in the absorption of Vitamin D, is also important for bone formation. Studies show that zinc supplements can slow bone loss and boost immunity. Most supplements contain the recommended dosage of zinc.

Boron

This trace mineral assists calcium and magnesium metabolism; a deficiency can affect proper bone and joint function. The recommended intake is 12 to 18 mg per day, which is typically the level found in a good multimineral supplement. When you take zinc, copper needs to be taken with it in a ratio of 10-15 parts zinc to one part of copper. If you do not get the needed copper, you may develop a copper deficiency—with a chance of developing weakened blood vessel walls or copper deficient anemia.

Folate

Folate, as mentioned previously, lowers homocysteine by acting as a cofactor in the recycling of methionine. Folate blocks xanthine oxidase, an enzyme involved in the conversion of purines into uric acid. Folate deficiencies can cause a type of anemia in which the red cells become few, too large, and pale (a macrocytic, hypochromic anemia). Folate is a serotonin booster. Since it's a water-soluble vitamin, it's easy to develop folate deficiency, which can, among other things, contribute to depression. Estrogen and progesterone replacement can deplete folic-acid levels. The birth-control pill depletes folic-acid levels. Take at least 800 mcg daily, which will also lower your homocysteine level and protect against hardening of the arteries.

Vitamin E

Vitamin E gets a lot of press for its antioxidant and heart-health benefits. It also has been proven to be an excellent supplement for general menopausal support. Women who take vitamin E on a consistent basis have reported relief from hot flashes, night sweats, dry skin, vaginal dryness, and breast tenderness.

Since vitamin E is fat-soluble, take it with food for proper absorption. Many antioxidant vitamin/mineral formulations contain vitamin E, but you can also take it separately. The recommended dosage is 200 IUs one to three times daily. Individuals with diabetes, hypertension, or a rheumatic heart condition should not exceed recommended dosages. Since vitamin E has the potential side effect of raising blood pressure, women with hypertension or a family history of high blood pressure should consult with a health-care provider prior to using it.

Vitamin B$_6$

Vitamin B$_6$ is involved in hundreds of bodily functions, including dopamine production, the manufacturing of amino acid, and hormone regulation. For menopausal women, it can help alleviate bloating and water retention, diminish mood swings and anxiety, and regulate appetite and sleep. It is also a cofactor in turning dietary tryptophan into serotonin. Without enough B$_6$ in your body, you may develop depression.

Many adults are deficient in Vitamin B$_6$. The recommended dosage is 50 to 100 mg daily, as part of a B-complex vitamin supplement. It's also important to note that estrogen and progesterone replacement can deplete folic acid and B vitamins, including B$_6$.

In a sense, in order to optimize health in menopause all of the essential vitamins and minerals need to be present in adequate amounts. I recommend to all of my patients to take a quality, bioavailable vitamin, mineral and plant derived trace mineral supplement along with essential fatty acids. This provides all the essential nutrients as well as the targeted essential vitamins and minerals described above.

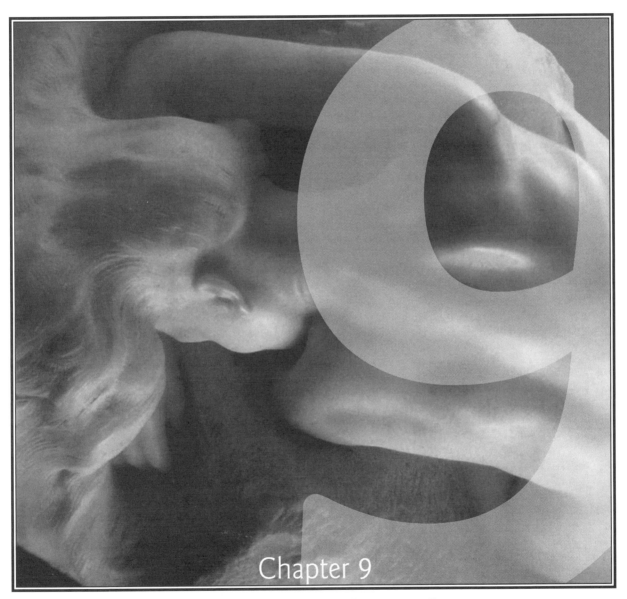

Chapter 9

Exercising for Life

Chapter 9
Exercising for Life

Keeping fit by exercising on a regular basis is one of the most important things that women of all ages can do to protect their good health. For women in their menopausal years, it's especially vital. Not only can a regular exercise program ease many of the symptoms associated with menopause, such as depression, weight gain, irritability, insomnia, and loss of concentration, but it can also help reduce the increased risks of heart disease and osteoporosis.

Sadly, the majority of women in the United States—60 percent, according to some research—don't get regular exercise or enough exercise to meet the established guidelines for health benefits, which is 30 minutes or more of moderate-intensity activity on most days, if not every day, of the week. There are a number of reasons for this, ranging from time and financial constraints to lack of motivation and energy.

If you're one of the 60 percent of women who don't regularly exercise or don't get enough exercise, know that it can be easier to incorporate health-boosting exercise into your daily schedule than you think. You'll find out how to do it, as well as learn more about the reasons why you should, in this chapter.

The Active Woman

Women were born to be active, and they have been so since the dawn of history. When the men were out hunting, women shouldered the main responsibilities for providing the other foods for their tribes. They worked the fields and gathered foodstuffs in the wild. In fact, women were the original beasts of burden when it came to ensuring the survival of their families. They stayed fit because they had to. It was a natural byproduct of their day-to-day existence.

Women today have more opportunities to

be active than ever before. However, the key word here is "opportunities." Unfortunately, all that our modern lifestyles offer us—both men and women—often results in disincentives to keeping fit. Yes, we have timesaving conveniences, but the time we save typically goes to something other than physical activity. The time saved driving to the grocery store could be spent doing some moderate-intensity physical activity when we get home. The problem is that we're more likely to park ourselves in front of the computer or the television with a snack than take the dog for a walk.

Women in general are less active than men. Why? There are a variety of reasons but the ones mostly commonly given are the following:

- not enough time
- can't afford it
- too many responsibilities at home and work
- health concerns
- don't know how to begin
- don't have the energy
- lack of motivation
- lack of the right equipment or access to it
- safety concerns
- don't know how to do it "right"

This last concern is especially troublesome. While there are guidelines for exercising healthily, there is really no right or wrong way to simply be active. Yet too many women let their concerns about not exercising "correctly," or their concerns about how they look when they do exercise, hold them back from doing things that could have a profound effect on their health, both now and in the future.

Keeping fit simply feels good. There isn't a body system that doesn't respond positively to exercise in some way. While the physical benefits of exercise, such as having lower body-fat levels and greater lean-tissue and bone mass, are often touted, exercise also has a profound effect on the psyche. Physical activity releases endorphins, which are the neurotransmitters that affect mood. Individuals who exercise on a regular basis are less likely to feel depressed, have a more positive outlook on life in general, and are better able to manage the stressors in their lives. Exercising regularly makes us feel good.

One study of more than 1,600 women found that sedentary women were twice as likely as their physically active counterparts to report hot flashes. In another, researchers reported that women experienced fewer hot flashes immediately following a 45-minute workout.

Exercise and Menopause

Keeping physically fit is especially important for women during their menopausal years. The benefits of a consistent exercise program are many, including the following:

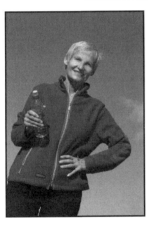

▸ Weight control. Women typically reach their maximum body weight during menopause, with an associated increase in body fat, which can contribute to heart disease and arthritis, among other health concerns. Studies show that women who are physically active during menopause are better able to keep their weight within normal ranges, have better fat to lean ratios, and can actually lose rather than gain weight during this period.

▸ Decreased heart-disease risk. Both moderate and vigorous exercise can lead to substantial reductions in the risk of heart attacks in postmenopausal women—in fact, the risk of incurring a heart attack decreases <u>50 percent</u> with regular activity. Exercise has also been proven to have a positive effect on cholesterol levels, increasing good cholesterol (HDL) and decreasing the overall cholesterol/HDL ratio.

▸ Stronger bones. Bone loss begins at around age 35, with women losing an estimated 1 percent of their bone mass per year. At menopause, the rate of loss accelerates to about 4 percent to 5 percent per year in the first five postmenopausal years. Weight-bearing aerobic exercise and progressive resistance training both slow bone loss and strengthen lean-tissue and muscle mass, which can protect against falls and fractures.

▸ Better blood-sugar levels. Regular aerobic exercise releases glucagon that is stored in the tissues into the bloodstream, which helps keep insulin levels down.

▸ Better hormone levels. Hormone levels—including estrogen levels—are typically better balanced in women who get regular exercise.

▸ Fewer vasomotor problems. Exercise

lowers the amount of circulating FSH and LH, which can trigger hot flashes. It also raises endorphin levels, which drop during a hot flash. Regular exercise has been shown to decrease the frequency and severity of hot flashes in postmenopausal women.

▸ Improved mental functioning. Exercise improves the circulation in the body, including the circulation in the brain, and can positively affect cognition. It may also slow the loss of dopamine, which helps prevent the shaking and stiffness that often accompany aging.

▸ Better, more restful sleep. As little as 20 minutes of moderate aerobic exercise a day can promote better sleep patterns and more restful sleep.

▸ Fewer mood swings and less depression. Exercise promotes good mental health and a positive mood state. Menopausal women who exercise regularly say they have an easier time dealing with stress and are less depressed in general.

Regular exercise has also been shown to have a positive affect on reducing the risks of certain types of cancer, including the breast and endometrial varieties.

Time to Get Moving!

What's the best kind of exercise? Most people find that simply walking vigorously is easiest, most convenient, and least likely to cause injuries. Everyone knows how to walk, and all you really need is a good pair of shoes and some comfortable clothes to get started. But walking isn't the only option open to you. Walking, running, aerobic dance (and other forms of dance), jumping rope, working out on a treadmill, and bicycling are all good choices.

To reduce your risk of osteoporosis, choose activities that require the use of the hips and legs. Weight lifting or resistance training, which stresses the bones in a different way, is also good for reducing bone loss.

> According to the North American Menopause Society (NAMS), high-impact exercise, such as running, step aerobics, and gymnastics, provides the greatest bone-building benefits.

The good news about exercise is that it's not necessary to "go for the burn." You can if you want, but numerous studies have shown that exercise that pushes your heart rate up to a moderate exertion level—60 percent to 85 percent of your maximum heart rate (an estimated 220 beats per minute)—is just as effective.

There are a number of maximum-heart-rate calculators available free on the Internet. Just type "maximum heart rate calculator" into a search engine.

How much exercise do you need? Probably not as much as you think. Walking as little as a mile a day has been shown to reduce the risk of osteoporosis. In a study of 25,000 Norwegian women, researchers found that just four hours of exercise a week reduced the risk of breast cancer by 37 percent. Another study found that women who exercised for an hour three times a week increased their bone density by 2.6 percent in one year.

For heart health, guidelines published by the *Journal of the American Medical Association (JAMA)* recommend a total of 30 minutes or more of moderate-intensity physical activity on most, if not all, days of the week. However, you don't have to be active for 30 straight minutes if you don't want to be. Shorter bursts of eight to 10 minutes in duration have been shown to be equally effective.

How to Get Started

Regardless of what type of exercise you choose to do, it's a good idea to have a physical with a stress test first if you've been inactive for a while. Such testing is important for ruling out any undiagnosed medical problems that could affect your physical activity and is also valuable in establishing a baseline for measuring your progress.

Choose an activity or activities that you enjoy. Walking is the easiest and most convenient for most people, but it's not for everyone. If you find it boring, do something else. You'll be much more inclined to stick with activities that interest you than with ones that don't.

Whatever you do, do it at least three times a week for 30 minutes, at 60 percent to 85 percent of your maximum heart rate, which is 220 minus your age. As an example, a 45-year-old woman's maximum heart rate would be 175 (220 minus 45) and her exertion range (target aerobic heart rate) would be 105 to 149 (175 multiplied by 60 and 85 percent, respectively).

Start slowly and build gradually. Keep your workouts short at first and increase your sessions by just a few minutes each week. Be sure to start each workout slowly as well to allow your muscles and joints time to warm up. Don't stretch cold muscles. The best way to loosen them up is slow, easy activity. Stretching, however, should be a part of your post-workout cool down.

Wear comfortable clothing that is appropriate for your chosen activity. If you're exercising outdoors, use sunscreen and a protective hat if necessary. In cold weather, dress in layers that you can peel off if you get too warm. Keeping your head covered will also help you stay warm.

Hydration is the key to a good exercise program. If you're working out at a moderate intensity—enough that you're sweating—it's a good idea to drink a cup of water fortified with minerals before and after you work out. You lose a lot of minerals through sweating. If you can, take sips during your workout as well.

Be sure to make resistance-training part of your exercise program. Aim for three times a week and one to two sets of 10 reps each that work the large muscle groups—arms (forearm flexors and extensors, deltoid, biceps, triceps), chest (pectoralis), shoulders (supraspinatus, upper deltoids, upper trapezius, rotator cuff), back (sacrospinalis, latissimus dorsi, upper and lower trapezius, quadratus lumborum, psoas) and legs (hamstrings, quadriceps, calf gastrocnemius). Choose weights that challenge your muscles. By the time you complete the second set, or are nearing completion, your muscles should feel tired. As your strength improves, adjust the weights or resistance accordingly.

Flexibility and balance are also important for women to maintain as they grow older. Both can easily be improved through a general exercise program. Something as simple as sitting on a fitness ball while doing upper-body work is a great way to challenge more muscle groups and improve balance. Flexibility and balance can be improved through such activities as yoga and tai chi, which I'll discuss in more detail in Chapter 10.

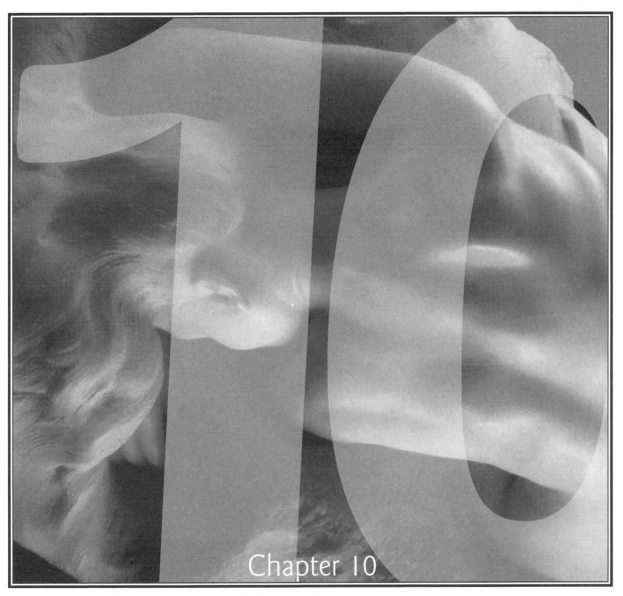

Chapter 10

The Mind/Body Connection

Chapter 10
The Mind/Body Connection

We live in a complicated world that grows more complex by the nanosecond. While modern technology has decidedly made many facets of life easier and more comfortable, in many respects it also complicates life beyond belief.

We are by no means the first generation to have to deal with stress, but today we're called on to cope with things that go far and beyond what our ancestors had to deal with. The pressures of commuting, raising families, being responsible citizens, holding down jobs, etc. can be overwhelming at times. For the conveniences and successes of our modern world, we often pay a huge price—and that price can come at the expense of our physical and mental health. In fact, stress along with stress-related complaints, is the leading reason behind trips to the doctor, accounting for an estimated 60 percent to 90 percent of all office visits.

Although there is still much to be learned when it comes to the complicated interactions that take place between our minds, our bodies, and the world around us, we do know that how we feel, both physically and mentally, is inextricably linked to many outside factors, some within our control and some not. When physical or mental problems arise, some form of drug therapy may be necessary; the most effective approach, however, includes taking these factors into consideration as well. This almost always means learning how to identify and cope with the things that cause stress in our lives and, by doing so, reducing our stress levels.

During the menopausal years, it's espe-

During the past decade or so, promoting health and recovery from illness through a variety of methods that enhance the natural healing capabilities of the mind and body, such as modern medicine, psychology, nutrition, exercise, physiology, nursing, and belief, has developed into what is now called mind-body medicine. Much of the pioneering work in this field has been conducted by Dr. Herbert Benson at Harvard Medical School, now also home to the Mind Body Medical Institute.

cially important to have a positive balance of energy uniting the mind, the body, and the outside world. The hormone fluctuations that take place during this time typically cause women to feel more irritable, more anxious, and more depressed than usual. Even women who are extremely well-balanced emotionally prior to menopause report changes in their moods that go beyond anything they experienced before, ranging from simply not feeling like themselves to feeling as though they no longer know the people inhabiting their bodies.

Changes in hormone levels also affect the autonomic nervous system, which controls respiration, pulse rate, glandular function, muscle tension, and blood circulation. When stress is added to the mix, the body can easily go into overload. The sympathetic nervous system responds to signals from the hypothalamus by releasing epinephrine and norepinephrine (and some other related hormones) causing heart and pulse rates to soar, muscles to tense up, blood vessels to constrict, and the person's breathing rate to speed up—all the classic elements of the "fight or flight" response that has protected human life from the earliest of times.

Today, these responses tend to kick in far too often. As they do, they contribute to numerous stress-related problems, including headaches, joint pain, cardiac disorders, chronic pain, fatigue, diabetes, and stomach disorders. They have also been shown to contribute to hot flashes, sleep problems, headaches, and depression in menopausal women. Learning how to reduce stress helps us better cope with the triggers to these responses, and have been shown to have a profound effect on our attitudes and our general health.

Stress reduction typically takes several forms, including restructuring your environment to make it less stressful and learning

If for any reason you feel the issues you're dealing with are beyond what you feel comfortable addressing on your own, I strongly encourage you to seek professional help. Getting a referral from your personal physician is often easiest, but you can also contact professional organizations (you'll find several pertinent ones listed in the resource section) for help in locating a qualified professional in your area. Another possible approach is to look for women's clinics that offer counseling services or support groups for women approaching or in menopause.

relaxation and stress-reduction techniques to evoke changes in your behavior or physiology. Many of the common approaches in both areas are easy to learn on your own. However, it's sometimes necessary to seek the help of a qualified professional for counseling or coaching.

There are a number of different relaxation and stress-reduction techniques to choose from, including yoga, meditation, massage, breathing exercises, listening to music, you name it. Some people find light exercise to be extremely calming. Even something as simple as changing the colors in your home or office can contribute to a less stressful environment. You can sit zazen like the Buddhists do, have acupuncture treatments to balance your chi, meditate to remain calm, pray for serenity, or practice qi-gong to learn to control your own healing energies; you name it. The goal is to do what you need to do to relax and thereby foster an environment of peace and calm.

Following are some introductory descriptions of some of the more popular relaxation approaches. As you read through them, you'll probably find some that you're familiar with and others that you might like to try. Keep in mind that what works for others may not

According to a study conducted by the North American Menopause Society, 25 percent of women have used some type of relaxation therapy, such as meditation or yoga, to relieve their menopausal symptoms.

A 2003 survey by the National Centers for Disease Control found that 46% of the women they surveyed had used complementary or alternative therapy either alone or in combination with conventional therapies for relief of their symptoms.

work for you and that you might have to try a few different approaches to find the ones that fit best for you.

Whatever approach you take, it's a good idea to find something that will allow you to take a 20-minute relaxation break every day. Many of the following techniques can also be employed as "mini relaxations" and used when necessary during times of stress.

Deep Breathing/Paced Respiration

Controlled deep breathing can dramatically improve how you feel by increasing oxygen flow to all tissues of the body. It helps relax the entire body, undoing the damage done by shallow, rapid breathing, and strengthens the muscles in the chest and abdomen.

The average adult will inhale and exhale about sixteen times per minute. Each time about a half a liter of air is inhaled and then exhaled. However, when we feel anxious we tend to take shallow frequent breaths from our chest. Deep breathing allows you to

In a study of 33 subjects, researchers at the Wayne State University School of Medicine found that women trained in paced respiration or deep breathing were able to cut the frequency of hot flashes by half. In another study, researchers at Harvard found that women who listened to a relaxation tape, which included guided imagery and breathing exercises, each day for 30 minutes reported that hot flashes were reduced by one-third.

increase the amount of air you are inhaling with each breath.

Tension-taming Deep-breathing Exercise

Stand with your fleet slightly apart and your arms hanging relaxed at your sides. Breathe in through your nostrils, allowing your lower abdomen to rise. As you breathe in, imagine the oxygen flowing throughout your body reaching all the way out to the tips of your toes and fingers. Breathe out noisily

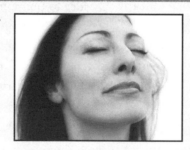

through the mouth, allowing your abdomen to fall. As you breathe out, imagine all the

tension and anxiety flowing out of your body onto the floor. Feel your muscles relax as you let go of the tension. Repeat several times until you feel relaxed. This is a great exercise to try in conjunction with other relaxation techniques.

Meditation

There are many different meditation techniques, but they all focus primarily on quieting the body by quieting the brain. During meditation, brain waves switch from fast beta waves to alpha or theta waves—the slower brain waves that lead to a calmer, happier state of mind. The body's metabolism slows down, with corresponding decreases in respiration and heart rate.

There are four basic elements that just about all styles of meditation share. They are as follows:

- a quiet location for the mediation to take place

- a comfortable posture

- an object to focus attention on (possibly a word or phrase)

- a passive attitude

You should try to find a quiet place with a minimum amount of distractions to practice meditating. As you get more comfortable with the practice, you will be able to call on your mediation skills to relieve tension whenever you need to—even in public settings with lots of noise and activity. You should develop a routine of meditating one to two times a day and stick to it. Women often tend to feel guilty about taking the time to "sit and do nothing," but remember that you are making an investment in your health.

Basic Meditation Exercise

Choose a quiet spot away from distractions like the telephone and television. Sit in a comfortable position. Pick a focus word or phrase that is important to you: "Peace," for example. Close your eyes. Become aware of your breathing. Starting at your forehead and working your way all the way down to your toes, relax each of your muscles. Imagine the tension from each muscle being blown out of your body with each outward breath.

Breathe in and out at your normal relaxed pace. With each outward breath, silently say your focus word.

Remain passive in your thoughts and don't worry about whether you are doing things "right" or about any outside issues. If you find your mind wandering back to conscious thoughts, simply let the thoughts go and return to the repetition of breathing and saying your focus word.

You should spend between 10 and 20 minutes meditating. (It is fine to check the time during your mediation session.) Take a few moments after you finish meditating to continue sitting quietly before you stand up.

Acupuncture and Acupressure

The techniques of acupressure and acupuncture originated thousands of years ago in traditional Chinese medicine. Both use pressure applied to specific points on the body to release and rechannel blocked vital energy, often referred to as "chi" or "qi." Traditional healers believe that an imbalance, or blockage, of energy is the root cause of all illness.

In acupuncture, hair-thin needles are inserted into specific areas of the body. In acupressure, the same areas are stimulated with pressure applied with the fingers or small metal balls.

Both practices stimulate the release of pain-relieving endorphins. They encourage the body to balance and heal itself while producing feelings of improved vitality and well-being. Stimulating specific points on the hands and feet may help balance hormone production and possibly reduce hot flashes, headaches, heavy or erratic menstrual bleeding, insomnia, and stress.

It is, of course, important to choose an acupuncturist carefully. Most states require that acupuncturists be licensed. The National Certification Commission for Acupuncture and Oriental Medicine can provide you with a list of certified practitioners in your area. Check the resource section at the end of this book for contact information.

Energy-upping Acupressure Exercise

Place your index finger between your eyebrows and apply gentle pressure to this spot for one minute. By stimulating blood flow to the brain you can restore energy and increase concentration levels.

In one 1994 trial of menopausal women, Swedish researchers reported that patients undergoing acupuncture for eight weeks experienced half the number of hot flashes they had felt before treatment, with the benefits of treatment extending for three months after it ended.

Stress-stopping Acupressure Exercise

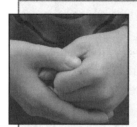

Place your hands on your tummy so that your fingers meet across your bellybutton. Gently press on this spot for a minute to calm your sympathetic nervous system, which is responsible for the release of the stress hormone cortisol.

Biofeedback

Biofeedback is a technique in which mechanical monitoring devices are used to provide feedback on body functions, such as heart rate and blood pressure, in an attempt to teach someone to voluntarily control certain body processes. This method helps teach patients to observe how their bodies respond to specific thoughts and situations, both positive and negative, so that they can then train themselves to control their bodies.

When you find yourself in a stressful situation, your pulse rate will automatically become elevated and your breath rate will increase. The opposite is true if you are in a particularly calm situation. Both your heart rate and your breathing slows down. These processes occur naturally. Through biofeedback, you may be able to control such processes and thereby rid yourself of bothersome symptoms such as headaches and hot flashes.

Several studies report that biofeedback that focuses on the physiology of the pelvic-floor muscles can help improve bladder control in some women. A device called a transvaginal sensor can be inserted into the vagina. The sensor is connected to a computer that monitors muscular activity and allows a woman to see if she is effectively contracting her pelvic muscles and not other muscle groups, such as those that involve the stomach or buttocks. Additional sensors may be placed in other areas, such as the inner thigh and abdomen to help a woman identify when she is not tensing the correct muscles. A typical biofeedback session lasts about 20 to 30 minutes, and usually about a dozen sessions are needed to get the best results.

If a woman is uncomfortable with this form of biofeedback, she can, of course perform kegel exercises, which have been shown to be very beneficial, on their own. In one Belgian study, published in the journal *BJU International*, researchers found that pelvic-floor-muscle exercises were successful in treating urinary incontinence in over half the women they tested. In the group that the exercises were not found to be initially successful, another 24% reported significant improvements during the 10-year follow-up to the study. Researchers concluded that 66% of women who have favorable results with kegel exercises have those favorable results persist for at least 10 years.

Kegel Exercises

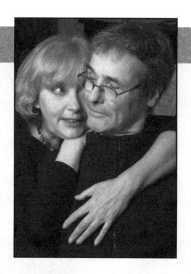

Kegel exercises are designed to strengthen the muscles in the pelvic floor. Many women who are experiencing minor urinary incontinence during and after menopause find that strengthening these muscles corrects or reduces the problem significantly. A bonus is that many women find the exercises make the vaginal muscles more sensitive and report increased sexual pleasure.

Kegel exercises are very simple to perform. Begin by trying to stop your flow of urine. The muscles you use to do this are the muscles you will be targeting. Once you have identified those muscles you will perform the exercises when you are not urinating.

❶ Tighten the pelvic-floor muscles and muscles around the rectum and hold for four seconds; then relax. Tighten and relax these muscles 10 times.

❷ Perform this exercise five to eight times a day.

Since no one will know you are doing the exercises you can perform them anytime such as when you're at your desk, while you're waiting in a grocery line, or while you're in the car. Many women report that they see a definite improvement after three to six months of faithfully doing these exercises.

Biofeedback is also often used to treat stress. By using sensors that measure skin temperature, skin electrical activity, and muscle electrical activity, some women can learn to control and calm their stress reaction.

Through the use of either a pen on a graph plotter or tones fed through headphones, a physical representation of the effectiveness of work being done is created.

Yoga

Yoga combines physical exercise with deep breathing and meditation. Regular practice promotes health on all levels—physically, emotionally, and spiritually. Yoga can improve blood circulation, help maintain muscle tone and flexibility, and increase levels of mood-regulating chemicals in the brain. As such, it can have a powerful effect on menopausal symptoms like insomnia, hot flashes, mood swings, and depression. It also provides weight-bearing exercise that encourages bone health. And, as anyone who regularly practices yoga can tell you, it can also be a good cardiovascular exercise, which can help lower your cholesterol level and improve cardiovascular health.

There are many different types of yoga, all typically combining breathing exercises, warm-ups, poses, and meditation. Hatha yoga, which is a combination of many different types, is the most common form practiced in the United States.

The best way to learn yoga is to take classes from a qualified instructor. If you don't have access to classes where you live, videotapes and DVDs are also valid methods of learning the practice. There are several organizations that require specific training standards of their members and may be able to make recommendations for qualified yoga teachers in your area. See the resource section at the end of this book for contact information for several of them.

Other Eastern Practices

Qi gong (pronounced "chee gung") is considered the primary form of therapeutic exercise in traditional Chinese medicine. It is actually an all-encompassing term that includes over 4,000 individual practices of exercise, meditation, and martial arts. Tai chi (pronounced "tie chee") is a martial art based on the principles of Qi gong. It involves deep breathing, meditative thought, and slow gentle movements that have been found to increase muscle mass and improve balance, thereby reducing the risk of osteoporosis.

In one 1996 study a group of seniors practiced tai-chi for 15 weeks and reduced their risk of multiple falls by a dramatic 47.5 percent. As a side benefit, members of the same group experienced reductions in their blood pressure by the end of the study as well. In a more recent study, published in March 2004, researchers at the University of Liverpool reported that tai chi was shown to significant-ly improve balance and blood pressure in middle-aged women. The *Archives of Internal Medicine* recently reported on a systematic review of the research on tai chi, confirming that it has both physiological and psychological benefits, promoting flexibility, balance, and cardiovascular fitness, for older patients.

There are five different recognized styles

Directions for Performing Tai Chi Movement:
Golden Rooster Stands On One Leg

Stand facing forward with your feet about a shoulder's length apart.

Relax your shoulders, wrists, and elbows, allowing your arms to hang at your sides with your hands open facing inward.

Take one step forward with your right foot and raise the heel slightly, allowing your weight to rest on the left leg (which should be slightly bent at the knee).

Slowly raise your right hand in front of you with the wrist relaxed and your palm down. At the same time, bend your left wrist downward and begin bending your left elbow so that it is parallel with your waist.

Bend your right elbow up so that your open hand faces forward, and at the same time lift your right leg, bending it at the knee (see picture), making your right thigh and your right upper arm parallel, You will now be balanced on your right leg.

Pause slightly; then lower your right arm and leg smoothly, returning them to the original relaxed position.

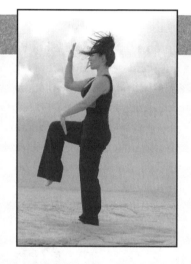

At the same time, lower your left arm back to its relaxed position at your side.

Repeat the entire set of movements several time and then switch sides, mirroring the movements on the left side as well.

of tai chi and many variations within those five groups. It has become increasingly popular, and classes can now often be found at local gyms, YMCAs, and Eastern-practice centers. Classes normally start with warm-up and breathing exercises and end with a cool down and perhaps meditation. Your instructor will demonstrate the individual movements step by step, and eventually you will learn to link the gentle movements into longer sequences.

13 Basic Principles of Tai Chi

There are a number of styles and variations of tai chi, but most of them adhere to the following basic principles.

1. Sink your shoulders and drop your elbows down.
2. Relax your chest and round your back.
3. Sink your chi, life energy force, downward.
4. Lightly point your head up.
5. Relax your waist and hips.
6. Be aware of yin and yang, like the difference between empty and full.
7. Coordinate the upper and lower parts of your body.
8. Use the power of your mind instead of using force.
9. Establish a harmony between the internal and the external.
10. Connect your mind and your chi (life force).
11. Find stillness within movements.
12. Allow movement and stillness to exist at the same time.
13. Always use continuity and evenness throughout the forms.

Reiki

Similar in some aspects to acupressure, the Japanese practice of reiki (pronounced "ray key") uses gentle laying on of hands to specific areas of the body to balance and direct energy, allowing the body to heal itself. Unlike the case with acupressure, however, there is no physical manipulation of the body. The client often experiences pleasant warmth from the practitioner's hands, and most people report feeling very relaxed, often falling asleep during a session. Some people report feelings of alternating heat and cold, tingling, pressure, waves of energy, or even nothing at all. Women who have found success with reiki in treating certain menopausal symptoms report stress elimination and a reduction in both the intensity and the frequency of their hot flashes, among other things.

Reiki falls into a category known in medical circles as therapeutic touch (TT). Therapeutic touch is widely accepted as having positive effects for patients. One recently concluded 2003 study, the largest ever published on therapeutic touch, found that TT promotes comfort, calmness, and well-being.

A practitioner of reiki must have completed the Level 1, or first-degree course, as well as the Level 2, or second-degree practitioner's course taught by a reiki master. The best way to find a reiki practitioner is by word of mouth. You may want to check for local "New Age" publications, which are often found for free in bookstores, coffee shops and grocery stores. You also may locate practitioners online. Be sure to question your practitioner about his or her training before you agree to a first session. Most practitioners will have a certificate, issued by the reiki master they trained under, to show you as well.

Hypnosis

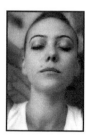

Hypnosis is a form of self-focused attention that can make it easier to relax or learn how to control bodily functions. It has been found to be useful in combating a number of symptoms associated with menopause.

A study published in the March/April 2003 issue of *Women's Health Issues* demonstrated that hypnosis significantly reduced the duration and severity of hot flashes. In addition, it was found to improve participants' sleep, resulting in reduced incidences of insomnia and significantly improved fatigue

levels. Participants reported a significantly improved overall quality of life as a result of the hypnosis sessions.

You can participate in group-hypnosis sessions guided by an instructor, work one-on-one with a hypnotherapist, or practice self-hypnosis. There are a number of books, tapes, and videotapes available for teaching yourself hypnosis. See the resources section for information on an online organization that can help with recommendations for a professional hypnotherapist in your area.

Self-hypnosis Exercise

Find a comfortable spot where you are unlikely to have any interruptions for at least 10 minutes. Sit in a comfortable position and decide what the intended focus of your hypnosis session is going to be, perhaps relaxation or reducing hot flashes. Direct your attention on a small object in the room and focus on your breathing. Breathe in through your nose and out through your mouth as you relax your entire body. Focus on the object, keeping your intended focus in the back of your mind. As you focus on the object and your intention, you will notice that your eyelids will become heavier. Allow them to close when it feels natural to do so. Allow the ideas and images that come to you to flow naturally. Begin to focus in on whatever emerges as most important in that moment. As you relax, allow yourself to experience your focusing and refocusing on whatever is important. At some point, you will feel your session moving towards a natural conclusion. Open your eyes when it feels natural to do so. Remain seated quietly for a few moments before rising. You will find that practicing self-hypnosis will allow you to enter into this relaxed state much quicker and with little effort.

Reflexology

Similar to shiatsu and acupressure, reflexology manually stimulates reflex points on the ears, hands, and feet to release and balance energy. Points that relate to the pituitary, thyroid, adrenals, solar plexus, and reproductive organs are commonly stimulated to relieve menopausal symptoms.

One randomized controlled study, published in 2002, found that both reflexology and foot massage reduced anxiety, depression levels, hot flashes, and night sweats in menopausal women. Another study, conducted by the Oregon Research Institute, a nonprofit behavioral research center, showed that the practice of cobblestone-mat walking, a reflexology

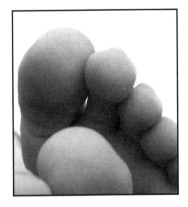

practice based on the cobblestone paths found in China, resulted in significant improvements in mental and physical well-being, including drops in blood pressure and reduced pain levels.

For information on organizations that certify and make referrals to qualified reflexologists in your area, see the resource section at the back of this book.

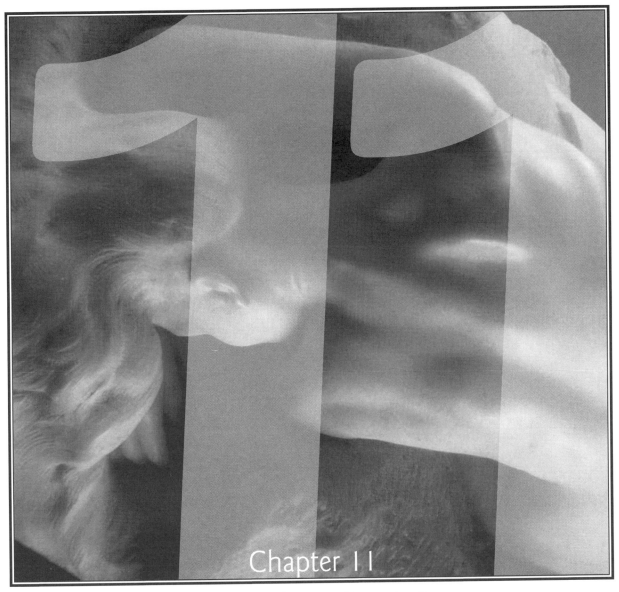

Natural Remedies for Menopause

Chapter 11

Natural Remedies for Menopause

Concerns over hormone replacement therapy have sent many women searching for other ways to manage the symptoms of menopause. It's also driven a growing market for products to meet their needs. Over the past few years, health-product manufacturers have brought a number of new products to market as alternatives to HRT. Walk into almost any retailer that carries dietary supplements (such as a health food store, a natural food store, a drug store, or even a big-box retailer) you're bound to see some products targeted directly to menopausal women. They're also widely available online.

While many of the products currently on the market are new, using plants to help control menopausal symptoms like hot flashes and vaginal dryness is anything but. Herbs like vitex were well known to ancient healers, including, by the way, Hippocrates, who prescribed it for menstrual problems. As you'll see in the descriptions of some of the herbs that follow, phytomedicine—or plant-based medicine—also plays a significant role in the medicine bag of indigenous peoples.

Although there is much that we still don't know about how herbal remedies actually work, we do know that many of the herbs traditionally used for women's health conditions contain phytoestrogens. As discussed in previous chapters, phytoestrogens and their metabolites can bind to estrogen receptors in the breast, in the uterus, and elsewhere in the body, thereby easing menopausal symptoms without increasing the risk of breast cancer. The jury is still out on the potential benefits of phytoestrogens and the best way to get them. They come in many forms. The most potent are compounds called isoflavones, which are found in high concentrations in legumes, especially soy, as well as in red clover and other herbs.

In fact, some experts think phytoestrogens have both estrogenic and

> Since 1934, more than 5,000 plants have been identified as containing substances with progesterone-like chemistry.

anti-estrogenic effects; that means they may even help prevent breast cancer by locking onto receptors in breast cells, keeping the body's own estrogen from locking onto the cells. However, this dual role of phytoestrogens has caused some experts to call for caution and more research when it comes to certain phytoestrogens and breast-cancer survivors' use of them. For example, genistein, a phytoestrogen found in many plant products, has been shown in some instances to both inhibit *and* stimulate the growth of some human breast-cancer cells. For this reason, some herbs might not be safe for women at risk for breast cancer or its recurrence. At this time, there is no research that can state definitively whether they are or not. As always, it is best to consult with a professional before taking any new supplement.

One stumbling block with alternative treatments like herbal remedies is that in the United States, because of funding issues, many have not been tested for efficacy and safety in large, placebo-controlled trials as pharmaceuticals are. However, a great deal of quality research does exist from studies conducted and published overseas, especially in Europe, Japan, and India. Combining this available international research with anecdotal

---

Results from a survey of 100 peri- or post-menopausal women at a San Francisco women's-health conference in March 2000 suggest that combining dietary supplements and HRT provided enhanced relief of certain menopausal symptoms.

Of the women surveyed, 29 percent used only HRT, 16 percent used HRT with dietary supplements, 32 percent used dietary supplements alone, and 13 percent used no product or used supplements excluded in the survey. The most common dietary supplements used were soy (29 percent), Ginkgo biloba (16 percent), and black cohosh (10 percent).

The women who used HRT alone reported significantly better relief of hot flashes than those who used dietary supplements alone (63 percent vs. 30 percent); however, perceived quality of life and overall control of menopausal symptoms were highest among women who used only dietary supplements and women who used combination therapy. Women using combination therapy also reported enhanced improvement in vaginal dryness, libido, and mood as compared with women using HRT alone.

---

reports and case studies creates a compelling argument for the use of herbal medicines for menopause.

The good news is that the interest in using phytomedicine to address a number of health concerns has been steadily growing in recent years. As a result, increasingly more studies are being conducted in the United States on herbal products. Many have shown great potential as alternative therapies and are gaining wider acceptance.

According to the North American Menopause Society, one-in-10 women uses herbs to ease menopausal symptoms.

Understanding the Dietary-supplement Industry

Along with the increasing interest in and acceptance of dietary supplements has come an increase in the confusion surrounding them. Understanding a little bit about how the dietary-supplement industry works and is regulated can help you make more informed choices. In the United States, herbal remedies are classified as dietary supplements. They are defined by law as products that contain one or more of the following dietary ingredients:

- a vitamin
- a mineral
- an herb or other botanical
- an amino acid
- a dietary substance used to supplement the diet by increasing the total daily intake

- a concentrate, metabolite, constituent, extract, or combination of these ingredients

Supplements are regulated to a certain extent, but they do receive less scrutiny than what prescription drugs go through. Manufacturers must follow certain regulations to produce and market dietary-supplement products. But, while they *are* responsible for ensuring that the products they make or distribute are safe and that any claims or representations made about those products are not false or misleading, they don't have to prove that their products provide specific benefits. Also, the amounts of active ingredients in a specific supplement can vary widely depending on the company producing them. This makes it all the more crucial for consumers to consult with well-educated nutritionally oriented physicians in making supplementation choices in the treatment of menopause and other conditions.

Only choose products made by reputable manufactures that you feel you can trust. A legitimate manufacturer should be happy to provide you with detailed ingredient listings on his websites or upon request.

Be an educated consumer. Learn as much as you can about the ingredients in any supplement you are considering. Nutritionally oriented physicians or herbalists are often the best professionals to consult in clarifying what is and what isn't a quality product.

Choosing Quality Natural Remedies as Supplements

No two supplements are alike when it comes to their ingredients. Because there are no specific standards set for what these products can contain, their efficacy, or what they can deliver, runs the gamut from highly effective to virtually worthless.

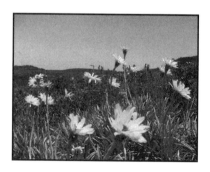

Natural remedies, and for that matter all supplements, may look extremely similar on the shelf, but they can differ greatly when it comes to what they'll do for you. For this reason, it's not the best idea to saunter into a store and grab the first product you see. It might be a good one. Then again, it might not be. The only way you'll be able to tell is by doing your research.

The product label will tell you some of what you need to know, including the following:

▶ the active ingredients in the product

▶ what form the ingredients take.

Herbal preparations should state the botanic name of the herb, such as Cimicifuga racemosa for black cohosh. Ideally, they should also state whether the herb is organically grown, wild crafted, or exactly how it is cultivated. When known and available, the active ingredient of the herb should be listed on the label and standardized for its active-ingredient content per serving; e.g. a 160-mg capsule of black-cohosh extract standardized to contain 4 mg of triterpenes per capsule.

Natural remedies present somewhat of a mixed bag when it comes to their use. It can be extremely difficult to separate hype from reality and figure out what works and what doesn't work from all the different treatments that are currently available. Furthermore, what works for one woman may not work for the next.

For these reasons, I highly recommend that everyone interested in using natural remedies do adequate research in this area. While cost isn't always an indication of quality in the supplement world, it is true in general that products that contain better ingredients will be more expensive than those that don't.

Before jumping on the bandwagon for a particular product, check out the research that backs it up. This is often available by going to the manufacturer's Website. If research isn't available on the Website, call and ask for it. A solid nutritional company will be able to send you this information. But be aware that supplement producers will not be able to discuss their products use over the phone.

It is always a good idea to exercise caution when using herbal remedies, especially if you're prone to allergic reactions. Before taking any product that's new to you, be sure to read the label carefully. If it contains ingredients that are unfamiliar to you, consult a good natural-medicine encyclopedia for any interactions or side effects that may affect you.

While most herbs are available either as single-herb preparations or in combination with other herbs, the jury is still out on whether one formulation is better than the other. The thinking behind combination herbal products is that if certain herbs individually are beneficial, combining them into one formula may be better. It's also believed that combining various herbs may deliver better results because of synergies between the various components of the herbs. On the other

If you don't have enough time to research products, or feel uncomfortable doing so on your own, find a health-care professional, preferably someone who specializes in natural medicine, who knows about these products and can advise you on what might work for you. Two possible sources for help in locating an alternative doctor in your area are the American Association of Naturopathic Physicians at www.naturopathic.org and the American College for Advancement in Medicine's Website at www.acam.org.

hand, it is sometimes difficult to figure out if combination herbals have sufficient amounts of any one herb to have a medicinal effect.

There are several studies that support the use of combination therapies. In one, women who took the supplement ArginMax for Women, which contains ginseng, Ginkgo biloba, the amino acid L-arginine, and 14 other vitamins and minerals, reported significant improvements in sexual desire and satisfaction as compared with women taking a placebo. Notable improvements were also made in the reduction of vaginal dryness, frequency of sexual intercourse and orgasm, and clitoral stimulation. At the same time, no side effects were reported.

Another study, reported on in the *Journal of Alternative and Complementary Medicine* in June 2003, confirmed the effectiveness of a combination morning/evening menopause formula. (Morning capsules contained Panax-ginseng, black cohosh, and soy and green-tea extracts, while evening capsules contained black cohosh, soy, kava, hops, and valerian extracts.) By the end of the second week of treatment, hot flashes were reduced by 47%. By the end of the eighth week, vasomotor scores were reduced by 50%, anxiety scores were reduced by 56%, and depression scores

were reduced by 32%. Overall sleep quality was also significantly improved.

If you're going to use combination products, read labels carefully and choose products that have better-known herbs, such as black cohosh and red clover, listed as main ingredients. If one herbal combination doesn't deliver the results you're looking for, experiment with other formulations or try products based on single herbs instead.

Black Cohosh

Botanical name: Cimicifuga racemosa. It's also known as bugbane, squawroot, rattle root, black snakeroot.

Currently one of the star alternative treatments, and the one that is probably the most talked about, black cohosh is a tall, flowering woodland plant that grows in forests from Ontario to Arkansas. It is no stranger to Native American medicine, where it is used to treat menstrual problems, pain after childbirth, nervous disorders, constipation, fatigue, and joint pain.

Black cohosh has also been used for more than 50 years in Europe to treat hot flashes, depression, and sleep disturbances. In Germany, the herb is endorsed by the

German Commission E, a government panel that reviews herbal remedies, for treating menopausal symptoms, including hot flashes and vaginal dryness. In fact, the journal *Alternative Therapies in Health and Medicine* reported that a number of clinical studies using Remifemin, a standardized black-cohosh extract, have shown that black cohosh is effective for the relief of some menopausal symptoms. Studies in the United States also confirm its value as an alternative treatment for these symptoms.

Black cohosh contains phytoestrogens. It also lowers luteinizing hormone (LH), which is thought to be one cause of hot flashes. New research also suggests that it may have some antioxidant properties. A study published in the journal *Maturitas* in March 2003 not only adds to the evidence of its effect on hot flashes but also hints at possible antidepressant activity. Some studies have found that black cohosh does not bind to estrogen receptors and has no estrogenlike activities, which could make it safe for women concerned about estrogen-related cancer.

How to take it: Look for capsules, tablets, or tinctures containing extracts standardized to contain 2.5% of triterpenes, the active ingredients in black cohosh. Black cohosh is sometimes sold as Remifemin.

For menopausal symptoms, take 40 to 160 mg of black cohosh daily. To reduce the chance of stomach upset, take it with meals. It can take four to eight weeks before you feel the benefits of taking black cohosh. Some experts recommend a six-month limit on taking the herb, but recent studies suggest that longer use is safe and free of significant side effects.

Cautions: Black cohosh has been shown to have few and mild side effects. It may cause stomach upset in certain people. One study suggested that it might induce slight weight gain and dizziness in certain women. It may also lower blood pressure. A very-high dose can cause nausea, vomiting, reduced pulse rate, heavy perspiration, headaches, and dizziness. Black cohosh contains salicylates; do not use it if you're sensitive to aspirin. Do not confuse it with blue cohosh, which is used for entirely different purposes and may cause significant side effects.

Chasteberry

Botanical name: *Agnus castus*. Also called Vitex and chaste tree.

Chasteberry is the fruit of a small Eurasian tree; however, both the berries and the leaves of the tree are used in chasteberry products. It is often used for treating PMS and for treating menopausal symptoms like hot flashes, sweating, vaginal dryness, mild depression, and irregular perimenopausal bleeding. Chasteberry was well known by many ancient healers, including Hippocrates, for example who wrote: "If blood flows from the womb, let the woman drink dark wine in which the leaves of the Vitex have been steeped."

The study most often cited on chasteberry was done in Germany in 2000 and involved more than 1,500 women ages 13 to 62, all with gynecological complaints. They were dosed with 40 drops of a commercially produced chasteberry product for an average of 166 days. Both patients and physicians reported 90 percent relief from fluid retention, breast tenderness, headaches, bloating, and fatigue after one month.

In a more recent study, the results of which were published in the journal *Complementary Therapies in Nursing and Midwifery* in 2002, chasteberry (Vitex) was found to give strong symptomatic relief of common menopausal problems. A round of follow up trials completed in the summer of 2002, and again reported on in the journal *Complementary Therapies in Nursing and Midwifery*, supported the initial findings that

Vitex oils are effective for the relief of menopausal symptoms.

How to take it: You can take either capsules that contain 200 to 225 mg of the crushed, dried fruit, standardized to contain 0.5% to 1.1% agnusides once or twice a day or 40 drops of extract with the same percentages of agnusides in one glass of water once a day. Chasteberry is often included in combination supplements. If you're using a product that contains it, go by the manufacturer's dosage recommendations.

Cautions: Excess use may cause itching, rash, stomach upset, headaches, or nausea.

Dong Quai

Botanical name: Angelica sinesis. Also known as Chinese Angelica, dang gui, and tang kuei.

Native to China and Japan, dong quai is a tall perennial herb that grows wild and is also cultivated for medicinal purposes. The rhizome of the plant is used in cooking. In traditional Chinese medicine, it is combined with other herbs for maintaining uterine health and regulating the menstrual cycle. As it contains phytoestrogens, it may also be useful for relieving hot flashes. Some of Dong quai's effectiveness may lie in the fact that it contains coumarins, which thin blood, dilate blood vessels, increase blood flow, and stimulate the nervous system.

Coumarins also appear to reduce inflammation and muscle spasms, which may account for dong quai's ability to reduce the severity of menstrual cramps. Other claims for the herb include correcting abnormal bleeding patterns, alleviating PMS symptoms, and improving vaginal dryness often associated with menopause.

Most of the studies on dong quai have been conducted in China and are of uncertain quality, which leads some experts to question the efficacy of this herb. Another reason why dong quai is difficult to assess is because it's often taken in combination with other herbs. The phytoestrogens found in dong quai may bind with estrogen receptors in cells minimizing some of the potentially negative effects associated with a woman's own estrogen, such as increased risk of breast cancer. One isolated study of particular concern, however, showed that dong quai might stimulate the growth of MCF-7 cells, associated with breast cancer. Most studies underscore dong quai's safety but question its ability to alleviate menopausal symptoms when used by itself instead of in combination with other herbs, as is done tradi-tionally in Asia.

How to take it: Dong quai is available in either pill or tincture form and is often combined with such other menstrual-cycle-regulating herbs as chasteberry, licorice, and Siberian ginseng. In either form, extracts should be standardized to contain 0.8% to 1.1% ligustilide, the active ingredient in dong quai. In pill form, take 600 mg of dong quai daily. In liquid form, take 30 drops (1.5 ml) of tincture three times daily. Continue taking dong quai for at least two months to see if it works.

Cautions: Be sure to buy Chinese or Japanese angelica (Angelica sinesis or A. acu-tiloba). Be careful about sun exposure when taking dong quai, as it contains compounds called psoralens that can make some people more sensitive to sunlight. Other possible side effects include a mild laxative effect, skin rash-es, and heavy menstrual bleeding.

Evening-primrose Oil

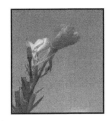

Botanical name:
Oenotheria biennis

The evening primrose plant is a wildflower native to America and is, so named for the late-afternoon opening of its flowers. The seeds of the plant are among the best natural sources of gamma-linolenic acid (GLA), an essential fatty acid from the omega-6 family.

The GLA in evening-primrose oil metabolizes into prostaglandins in the body, which helps control inflammation. For that reason it is widely used in Europe to treat diabetic neuropathy, mastitis, and eczema.

Studies have shown that evening primrose's anti-inflammatory properties might lessen breast pain associated with premenstrual syndrome. There isn't much clinical evidence to support its use in alleviating menopausal symptoms. In one trial that evaluated its effect on hot flashes, there was no discernable difference between evening-primrose oil and a placebo. However, there is strong anecdotal support for its use in lessening such symptoms as mood swings, anxiety, irritability, fluid retention, headaches, irregular bleeding, and vaginal dryness. For that reason, it is often included as part of a complete course of treatment for menopausal symptoms.

How to take it: The typical dosage is 1,000 to 1,500 mg twice a day for perimenopausal symptoms. It can take four to six weeks before discernible effects are realized. Maximum bene-

fits might take four to eight months to develop. Take with food to maximize GLA absorption.

Cautions: Evening primrose may cause bloating or gastrointestinal distress and is best taken with food. Do not use it if you are taking phenothiazine antipsychotics, have been diagnosed with schizophrenia, or if you are being treated for epilepsy.

Gingko biloba

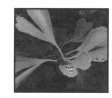

Botanical name: Gingko biloba. Also known as maidenhair tree and bai guo.

Gingko biloba is one of the oldest herbal remedies known to mankind. It is believed that it was first used in China around 2800 B.C. to treat breathing problems and enhance brain function. Many trials have underscored it's positive effects on boosting blood flow and increasing brain function, especially in the elderly. Thus, it may help alleviate such menopausal symptoms as forgetfulness, depression, anxiety, and headaches, all of which can be caused by reduced blood flow to the brain.

How to take it: Look for a supplement or extract that contains 24% flavones and 6% terpene lactones. Take 40 to 80 mg three times a day.

Cautions: Mild nausea and blood-pressure problems have been reported. Avoid use with other blood thinners, such as aspirin, heparin, and coumadin. Ginkgo biloba can affect insulin secretion and alter blood-glucose levels; individuals on insulin should consult with a doctor before using it. Adverse reactions are rare but have been reported with it has been used in combination with certain drugs, such as trazodone and prochlorperazine.

Kava

Botanical name: Piper methysticum. Also called kavakava and kawa.

Kava is a Polynesian evergreen shrub that is a member of the pepper family. The root of the shrub contains kavalactones, kava's active ingredient, which are known for their ability to relieve anxiety and induce sleep. Drinking kava is a part of many indigenous Polynesian ceremonies, where it is known as the "intoxicating pepper," and it has been compared to the use of wine in Western cultures.

Kava has been used for some time outside of Polynesia as an alternative to prescription tranquilizers and has been used extensively to lessen anxiety and insomnia. Unlike other traditional sleep remedies, kava remains effective over time. It may be helpful in treating such menopausal symptoms as anxiety and sleeplessness.

A German study published in the journal *Phytomedicine* in November 2003 studied the effects of a kava extract vs. a placebo in a group of subjects diagnosed with neurotic anxiety. The results showed consistent advantages of the kava extract over the placebo on a number of psychiatric scales. Overall significant improvements in the general well-being of the patients who took the kava extract were reported.

How to take it: Look for products that contain extract standardized to contain at least 30 percent kavalactones. Take 250 to 500 mg up to three times per day. Do not take for more than three months without supervision by a physician.

Cautions: There are some reports of liver toxicity with high dosages of kava, but none reported at recommended doses. The reports are rare and may be due to contamination by certain vendors rather than liver toxicity directly due to the plant. Some of the reported cases involved people taking other drugs at the same time along with Kava. These other drugs could have contributed to the reported liver toxicity. However, anyone with liver disease or risk factors for it should avoid taking kava. Discontinue use 24 hours prior to surgery. In recommended amounts, kava can cause mild stomach upset in some people. Long-term consumption may turn the skin, nails, and hair yellow temporarily. If that happens, discontinue use. In rare cases, kava can also cause rashes and other allergic skin reactions.

Korean Ginseng

Botanical name: Panax ginseng. Also called ren shen, Chinese ginseng, and Asian ginseng.

Ginseng is a small perennial that grows in many parts of the world. Panax, or Korean ginseng, which grows in moist forests in northeast Asia, is particularly prized for its adaptogenic qualities—in other words, it is thought to adapt itself to the unique needs of the individual taking it and restores balance in the body.

Panax ginseng is probably the best-known Chinese herb and is, in fact, one of the most important herbs in traditional Chinese medicine. It has been used for more than 7,000 years to combat fatigue and stress, and its medicinal benefits have been widely studied. It has been shown to prevent vaginal thinning,

and it may help relieve fatigue, insomnia, and depression. However, it's important to note that one study showed that ginseng stimulates the growth of MCF-7 cells, associated with breast cancer.

How to take it: Dosage varies according to body weight but is typically 1,000 mg for women weighing less than 130 pounds, 1,500 mg for women weighing 130 to 160 pounds, and 2,000 mg for women over 160 pounds. It's best to divide dosages over the course of the day and to take it on an empty stomach before breakfast and dinner. Look for ginseng in 500-mg capsules for dosing ease.

Cautions: Panax ginseng can cause temporary mild breast tenderness. It can also lower blood-sugar levels; diabetics interested in using it should first consult with their doctors. Discontinue use at least one week prior to surgery. In rare cases, Panax ginseng thins blood and can cause vaginal bleeding in post-menopausal women due to its mild estrogenic effect.

Licorice

Botanical name: Glycyrrhiza glabra.

Licorice is another herb with a long history. It was used in ancient Greece to calm coughs and soothe stomachs, and it is also a main component in Chinese herbal medicine. Its medicinal properties are in the root, or rhizome, which contains a substance called glycyrrhizin. Licorice also contains plant estrogens and flavonoids.

Licorice has been well studied and has been found to have a mild estrogenic effect. Glycyrrhizin, its active ingredient, can also enhance immune-system activity and possibly help protect one from cancer. Licorice may also help prevent heart disease by helping to keep arteries clear. It may help minimize menopausal symptoms, such as irritability, headaches, bloating, and breast tenderness. Licorice has been shown to enhance the effects of cortisol, allowing it to remain circulating in the body for longer periods. This is the mechanism by which licorice reduces inflammation.

How to take it: Licorice is made into capsules, tablets, wafers, tinctures, and cream for therapeutic use. A form of licorice, DGL, or deglycyrrhizinated licorice, has had the glycyrrhizin removed and is available in capsules and chewable wafers for calming coughs and soothing stomach upsets. The one to use for menopausal symptoms is the one that hasn't had the glycyrrhizin removed.

Dosage: Take a standardized extract (200-250 mg) three times daily. (A powdered root should be 1,000-4,000 mg daily. If you take a solid extract take ¼ tsp. before each meal.

Cautions: Licorice can cause fluid and salt retention and it shouldn't be taken by anyone who has high blood pressure, since it can interfere with medication prescribed for it. Use with caution if you have diabetes.

Red Clover

Botanical name: Trifolium pratense

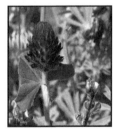

Red clover is a wild herb native to Europe, Africa, and Asia. It is part of the soy family and contains isoflavones and coumarins.

Traditionally, red-clover flower heads are made into a cough remedy for children and a topical treatment for rashes. However, red clover has also been shown to possibly be effective for treating hot flashes.

Most of the studies on red clover have been sponsored by Novogen, which manufactures a red-clover-based product called Promensil. The first U.S. study of Promensil was conducted at Tufts University in Boston, where 16 patients experiencing menopausal symptoms took it daily for two to three months. They reported a 56 percent decrease in hot flashes after eight weeks, along with a decrease in their intensity. There have, however, been conflicting studies on the herbs effectiveness.

Red clover might also protect against bone loss, according to a British study presented at the June 2000 meeting of the Endocrine Society. In the study, pre-, peri-, and postmenopausal women took one 40-mg tablet of Promensil for one year. The result was a 49 percent reduction in bone-mineral-density loss in the pre- and perimenopausal women.

How to take it: Take 400 to 500 mg of red clover, supplying about 40 mg of isoflavones, a day with meals. It may take four to five weeks to see results.

Cautions: None

Saint-John's-wort

Botanical name: Hypericum perforatum

Saint-John's-wort is a short, yellow-flowered perennial shrub that grows fairly easily in almost all soil conditions and is considered by some a noxious weed instead of a prized herb. It was well known to ancient healers and was one of the herbs prescribed by Hippocrates. St. John's Wort plays a key role in Native American healing as a mood enhancer and depression lifter. In Europe, the herb is widely prescribed for depression. It is not a prescription drug in the United States.

Although the herb's exact actions in the body are unknown, it contains hypericin and hyperforin; some experts believe these may act as serotonin reuptake inhibitors, causing nerve cells to retain more serotonin in their synaptic junctions. Some researchers believe it also functions as a monoamine oxidase (MAO) inhibitor, relieving certain types of depression.

It's effectiveness in treating mild-to-moderate depression is well-documented, with at least 25 double-blind clinical studies having been conducted. It's been found to be as effective as some prescription drugs in treating depression, with the added benefit of fewer side effects. Remember that certain prescription drugs act as serotonin reuptake inhibitors by using the fluorine molecule in their chemical structure to alter if not poison the nerve junction. Saint-John's-wort is also used to treat anxiety and sleep disorders. As such, it's of benefit to menopausal women experiencing these problems.

A clinical trial to investigate Saint John's wort's effectiveness in treating other problems specific to menopause was conducted in Germany in 1999. The results suggest that it does help relieve psychological and physical symptoms and enhance sexual well-being for menopausal women. More than three-quarters (76 percent) of study participants experienced significant lessening or disappearance of symptoms after 12 weeks of treatment.

How to take it: Saint John's-wort is available in a number of different formulations, including capsules, soft gels, tablets, tinctures, and creams. For best results, be sure the product you choose contains standardized extract containing 0.3% hypericin and hyperforin. For treatment of menopause symptoms, take 450 mg twice a day or 300 mg three times a day. Take with meals to avoid stomach upset. It may take four weeks to see effects. It may be taken indefinitely.

Cautions: Saint John's-wort can interfere with the actions of some drugs, including oral contraceptives and antibiotics. Adverse interactions have been reported between Saint John's-wort and indinavir, a protease inhibitor; and cyclosporine, a drug used to reduce the risks of rejecting organ transplants. Serious adverse reactions have been reported when combining Saint John's-wort with certain prescription antidepressants, such as Prozac and Zoloft. Side effects include dizziness, stomach upset, increased sensitivity to sunlight, dry mouth, and fatigue.

Valerian

Botanical name: Valeriana officinalis. Also called capon's tail and English valerian.

Valerian is a tall perennial herb native to Europe. The root and rhizome contain valeric or valerenic acid, a mild sedative. Its use dates back to the ancient Greeks and Romans. The Greek physician Dioscorides recommended valerian for a host of medical problems, including digestive problems, nausea, liver problems, and even urinary-tract disorders. It continues to be used extensively throughout Europe as a mild sleep aid and to reduce anxiety. Generally, it makes sleep more restful, helps people fall asleep easier and faster, and can be helpful for women who are experiencing sleep disorders during menopause.

Several clinical studies have found that valerian safely relieves occasional insomnia;

double-blind studies have found it to be more effective than a placebo and as effective as standard sleep medications for people with insomnia. Valerian is generally recognized as safe , is approved for food use by the FDA, and is approved by the German Commission E for nervousness and insomnia.

How to take it: Look for products standardized to 0.8 to 1.0% valerenic acid per dose. Dosage recommendations vary, but it's believed best to start with less and increase the dosage if necessary. Typical beginning dosages include 1 teaspoon of liquid extract in water or 400 to 450 mg 30 to 45 minutes before bedtime for insomnia. For anxiety, I recommend 1 teaspoon of liquid extract or 400 to 450 mg twice a day or as needed.

Cautions: Valerian has no known health hazards with recommended dosages. It may, however, impair the ability to drive or operate machinery and may interfere with central-nervous-system depressants. Some users report grogginess when they wake up. Use with caution with prescription sleep medications, tranquilizers, and antihistamines.

Wild Yam

Botanical name: Dioscorea villosa. Also called Mexican yam, devil's bones, rheumatism root, and colic root.

Wild yam is a climbing vine native to North and Central America, where it was used by the Aztecs and Mayans for pain relief. European settlers prized wild yam for its therapeutic properties in treating joint pain and colic. The root is the part of the plant that has medicinal value. It is available as a dried herb for use in tea and is also sold in capsule, soft gel, and tincture forms.

As noted in previous chapters, wild yam has been widely hailed as natural progesterone and a viable alternative to hormone replacement therapy. However, scientific studies have not yet supported these claims. While it does contain diosgenin, which can be converted to progesterone in a laboratory, eating wild yam or using products made from it has been shown to have little if any effect on menopause symptoms. There is, however, widespread anecdotal evidence for the use of it in relieving some menopausal symptoms.

An Australian study showed that short-term treatment with topical wild yam extract is free of side effects, but it appeared to have little effect on actual symptoms. In 1990, Dr. John Lee, a strong proponent of wild yam and natural progesterone derived from wild yam, documented, in a study of 100 women, its ability to increase bone density. Other studies have shown that the products don't consistently deliver hormone levels high enough to protect the uterus if the woman is on estrogen replacement therapy.

The North American Menopause Society does not support the use of over-the-counter progesterone creams; it recommends instead the use of prescription progesterone.

How to use it: If you decide to try "natural progesterone," ignore label claims about wild yam and bypass the dried herb and tinctures made from it. Instead, look for a cream that has been certified to contain 400 to 600 mg of USP-grade natural progesterone per ounce (28 grams), which will equal approximately 20 mgs of progesterone per gram (approximately ¼ of a teaspoon).

Apply about one-quarter teaspoon of the cream twice daily to large areas of relatively thin skin, such as the inner parts of thighs and arms, the face, the neck, your upper chest, and the abdomen. Rotate the site of application daily. It may take two or three months of use before maximum benefits are received. Skip one week of every month. It's usually easiest to time your skipped week with menstruation if you're still menstruating regularly. If you aren't, just schedule it on a calendar. When you are undergoing menopause, you may want to just continue to take the progesterone without discontinuing it. Please consult your physician.

Cautions: None are known for perimenopausal women. For postmenopausal women, using large amounts in excess of recommended dosages can cause spotting.

Homeopathy

Based on the principle of "like heals like," homeopathy uses minute amounts of substances derived from plants, animals, and minerals to cure symptoms that large amounts of these substances would normally cause in an individual. The remedies are formulated in tinctures or tiny pills.

Depending on the kind of symptoms a woman has, and her emotional, physical, and mental state, a homeopath can prescribe a number of different substances to treat menopause symptoms including the following:

▸ *Bellis perennis* for persistent backache and fatigue

▸ *Cimicifuga racemosa* for feelings of restlessness or mood swings

▸ *Sepia* for feelings of weakness or fatigue

▸ *Sepia* for heavy periods accompanied by bloating, depression, constipation, headaches, backaches or hot flashes

▸ *Sanguinaria* for heavy vaginal discharge, sore breasts, and right-sided headaches

▸ *Calcerea carbonica* for hot flashes

▸ *Belladonna* for excitability, restlessness, and vaginal dryness

In a small Polish study, 20 women taking a homeopathic remedy known as Feminon N for six months reported significant improvements in menopausal symptoms.

Homeopathic remedies are sold over-the-counter in health stores and some pharmacies. Many are single-ingredient formulations; however, also available are mixed homeopathic formulas that address a number of menopausal symptoms. (See the sidebar for an example of one such formula.) If you're considering using homeopathic products, consulting a trained practitioner to find the remedy best suited for your specific needs is <u>highly recommended</u>.

Spagyrism

There has been a renewed interest in an old form of homeopathic and herbal pharmacology known as spagyrism. First developed in the 16th century by the Swiss physician Paracelsus, spagyrism represents a form of homeopathy in which both vital healing energy and active substances are extracted from medicinal plants—creating powerful mother tinctures that can be made more potent by vigorously shaking them. Derived from the

Fem Estro HP® (formerly HP 3)

Fem Estro HP is an example of a high-quality, handmade homeopathic formula designed to address multiple menopausal symptoms , such as hot flashes, spontaneous sweats, tension, and anxiety.

Each drop contains the following:

Sepia officinalis	12 x
Sanguinaria canadensis	12 x
Sulphuric acid	6 x
Pulsatilla pratensis	12 x
Lachesis mutus	12 x
Lycopodium clavatum	6 x

Recommendation: For acute symptoms, dissolve 15 drops in your mouth every 30 minutes, reducing the frequency to three to four times daily upon improvement. Continue until your symptoms are relieved.

Form: a 1-fluid-oz. (30-ml)

Note: For more information on this product, see the resource section at the back of the book.

Greek words *spao* (separate) and *ageiro* (unite), the term spagyric means to take something apart and then reunite the parts.

Listed in the Homeopathic Pharmacopeia (HAB), the spagyric processing method produces medications with powerful energetic and biochemical effects. The combinations of spagyrically processed herbs, synergistic minerals, and homeopathic substances are designed to help the body eliminate toxins and restore proper physiological function.

One spagyric formulation designed specifically for treating menopausal symptoms, **Klifem**™, has been subjected to a study. Klifem is a mixture of Aletris farinose, Graphites, Helonias dioca, Pilocarpus microphyllus, Lachesis, Pulsatilla, Sanguinaria, and Larnium album. A multicenter clinical application study conducted by German physicians found that PEKANA's Klifem homeopathic-spagyric drops were effective in treating patients' menopausal symptoms, including hot flashes, night sweats, and mood swings. The survey, which involved a total of 67 female patients, investigated the medication for effectiveness, safety, and patient tolerance. More than 92 percent of the treating physicians and their patients reported that the drops were either very good (free of symptoms) or good (improved) in treating their symptoms. The phase IV study also confirmed that spagyric drops were free of side effects and well tolerated by more than 82 percent of their patients, even among women who required treatment for up to 12 months.

For more information on this product, see the resource section at the back of the book.

Women's Fx

Lydia Pinkims was a female missionary at the turn of the 20th century. She worked with Native Americans on their reservation, teaching them personal hygiene. Lydia noticed that the tribe she worked with was free of menstrual cramps, PMS and menopausal symptoms. In observing and talking with the women of the tribe, she discovered that all of the women in the tribe were taking certain herbs on a daily basis.

Ms. Pinkims saw this as a business opportunity and patented the formula, which she called Lydia Pinkim's Herbal and Vegetable Extract. The formula was often used by OBGYN medical doctors throughout the late 1950s. Unfortunately, however, once drug companies began marketing hormone replacement therapy and offering doctors financial kickbacks to prescribe it, use of Ms. Pinkims formula dropped off.

Women's Fx is a liquid reformulation that is an enhancement of the original Lydia Pinkims formula. Included in a 1-oz serving are a trace mineral complex: 250 mg, a pomegranate fruit concentrate (Punica granatum): 2,000 mg, a blueberry fruit concentrate (Vaccinum myrtillus): 2,000 mg, black cohosh (Cimicifuga racemosa – 2.5% triterpine glycosides): 75 mg, gamma oryzanol: 50 mg, green-tea leaf: 50 mg., soy isoflavones: 50 mg, and wild yam (Dioscorea villosa): 50 mg. It is recommended that the formula be taken twice a day.

See the resource section in the back of the book for more information on this highly bioavailable liquid formula.

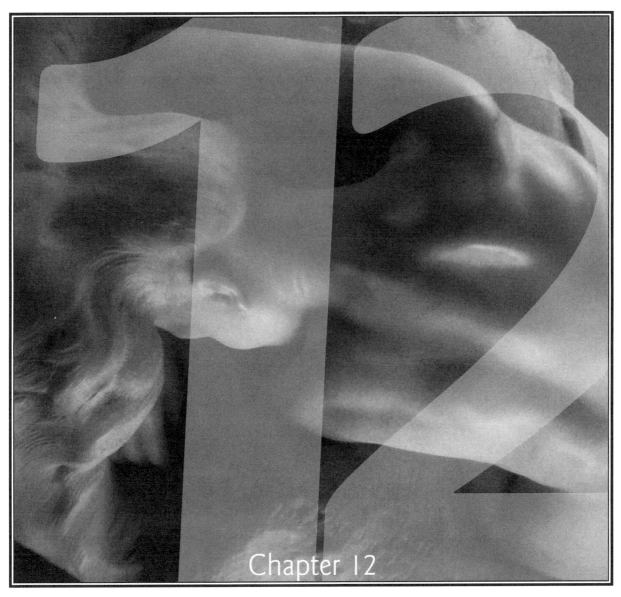

Chapter 12

Testing and Monitoring Your Hormone Levels

Chapter 12

Testing and Monitoring Your Hormone Levels

Throughout this book, I've stressed the importance of testing and monitoring hormone levels. One of the problems with conventional HRT is that it's often prescribed without the doctor's first assessing existing hormone levels. Furthermore, many women aren't consistently monitored when they're taking hormones. It's impossible to assess the effects of HRT without testing hormone levels on a regular basis, and it isn't possible to adjust dosages accurately without a clear picture of how each woman responds to the treatment.

All people react a bit differently to things that go into their bodies. With HRT, it's especially important to have an accurate read on what's going on inside you. In fact, it's vital. It's the only way to gauge whether the treatment you're receiving is really working.

Regardless of the approach you take to manage your menopause, it's important to commit to some type of testing on a regular basis. Doing so will help you avoid serious health problems in the future and put you into the most healthful state possible now.

Blood, saliva, and urine tests are all used for determining hormone levels. Each test has its supporters and detractors, primarily due to disagreements over the importance of testing for free, or available, hormones. These are hormones that have broken free from carrier proteins in the blood and that can freely enter target tissues.

Saliva tests measure free hormones and are an excellent way to assess hormone levels. Blood tests measure both the free and the inactive, or "bound," forms of hormones. They don't, however, always distinguish between the forms, and their results are less precise than those of saliva testing. Urine tests measure excreted hormones and/or their metabolites—not active, freely circulating levels. However, literature has well correlated excreted levels with free levels.

Blood Tests

Many M.D.s favor blood tests, which can measure both the total amount of estrogen, progesterone, and testosterone in the bloodstream and free, or unbound, levels. These tests are considered the gold standard when assessing women's-health issues in research settings. However, I and many other physicians don't feel that blood tests are up to par with saliva and urine tests—for the following reasons.

First, blood tests only can provide a one-time picture; that is, they only reflect the chemistry of the blood at the exact moment they are taken. Since hormones are released throughout the day, a single blood test can't accurately reflect fluctuations in their levels, which are affected by HRT drug metabolism, circadian rhythms, and other stressors.

Second, much of the hormone measured in blood tests is in bound form. It hasn't broken free from its carrier proteins and isn't in the form that the body can use. Some blood tests measure both the free and the inactive

forms of hormones, but they don't always distinguish between the two. For this reason, their result are less accurate than those that other types of tests provide.

Serum testing is also extremely expensive, which limits the number of hormones that can be affordably tested. Each hormone test can cost from $80 to $200. Tests for the free-serum levels of these hormones run $150 to $200 each. This makes comprehensive, integrated hormone monitoring unaffordable for most women. Typically, therefore, only estradiol and/or total estrogen is tested, because of the costs involved. Another factor is blood must be kept on ice in cool packs, which makes shipping costs high and increases the possibility of errors due to improper handling and storage.

While most results you see from research studies are based on blood tests, these tests must become much more affordable outside of clinical settings for them to be widely used. That said, some labs offer serum testing in combination with urine tests. Other labs enhance their serum panels by including SHBG (sex hormone binding globulin) while measuring all three hormones estrone, estradiol, and estrone along with their three metabolites 2,4, and 16 hydroxyestrone with progesterone, testosterone and DHEA. These comprehensive serum panels remain an excellent choice for monitoring hormone levels, as they measures hormones and their metabolites at an affordable price. See the resource section in the back of the book for more information.

Saliva Tests

Saliva tests measure unbound hormones. They are easy and inexpensive to perform and can be done anywhere and at any time.

Studies show a strong correlation between the levels of steroid hormones in saliva and free hormones in the bloodstream, which means that the amount of hormone found in saliva is an accurate reflection of hormone levels in the bloodstream.

The hormones found in saliva are in a stable form, which allows for great latitude in collecting samples. No special handling is required when shipping these tests.

The main drawback to saliva testing is that it can't be done on women who take hormones sublingually (under the tongue), as doing so can yield inaccurate results. Like blood tests, saliva tests only provide a snapshot of the hormone levels at the time at which the test is taken. Since, however, since

saliva tests are inexpensive, they can be taken more than once during the day.

Urine Tests

Twenty-four-hour urine tests, which measure excreted hormones and/or their metabolites, are the best way to evaluate hormone release throughout the day. These tests allow doctors and their patients to keep tabs on potentially carcinogenic estrogen metabolites.

The greatest disadvantage to 24-hour testing is that it measures only excreted hormones and/or their metabolites, not active, freely circulating levels. However, the medical literature has demonstrated correlated excreted levels with free levels. The test can also be somewhat inconvenient to perform, however, as they require saving all urine passed during a 24-hour period and keeping the urine refrigerated at all times. But these are minor annoyances when compared to the value of these tests.

If you can afford it, I recommend a blend of 24-hour-urine and serum-free-hormone level testing and/or sex binding hormone globulin levels (SHBG) if your physician offers them. While it's still expensive, the labs will normally bundle E1, E2, E3, with 2,4,16 hydroxyestrone, SHBG, progesterone, DHEA, and morning cortisol as a single panel and discount the total to make it affordable to you.

There are several excellent labs that can do these tests if they're not available where you live or if your health-care provider doesn't offer them. You'll find contact information for them in the resources section.

What Should Be Tested?

The best 24-hour urine tests will measure the primary and secondary steroid hormones and their most important metabolites, as listed below (list provided courtesy of Rhein Labs):

Estrogens

▸ estrone (E1)

▸ 2-hydroxyestrone

▸ 16a-hydroxyestrone

▸ 4-hydroxyestrone

▸ estradiol (E2)

▸ estriol (E3)

Androgens

▸ testosterone

▸ androsterone

▸ etiocholanolone

▸ androstanediol

▸ androstenetriol

▸ DHEA

▸ androstenedione

Progesterone

▸ pregnanediol (the primary metabolite of progesterone)

Corticosteroids

▸ cortisone

▸ tetrahydrocortisone

▸ corticosterone

▸ tetrahydrocorticosterone

▸ 5a-tetrahydrocorticosterone

▸ tetrahydro-11-dehydrocorticosteroine

▸ cortisol

▸ tetrahydrocortisol (THF)

▸ 5a-tetrahydrocortisol

Others

▸ pregnenolone

▸ pregnenetriol (5PT)

The best blood panels will include E1, E2, E3, 2-hydroxyestrone, 16 alpha-hydroxyestrone, progesterone, sex-hormone-binding globulin, DHEA, and testosterone. See the resource section at the back of the book for further information.

Menopause Case Histories

Following are two of the many menopause success stories that have come through our doors here at my clinic. They illustrate the individuality of this passage and the very real need for ongoing testing.

100 Years Young and Very Much "Kicking"

One of my favorite patients is M.B.H., who is currently 100 years young and will be celebrating her 101st birthday in 2005! Let's call her Ms. M. for short. Ms. M. has always been full of life and vitality, having taken many nutritional supplements for years. She has been postmenopausal for many years with a history of a heart murmur (mild aortic stenosis), some hypertension. and an enlarged left ventricle.

Our initial evaluation of her hormonal balance was performed with salivary testing in November 1998. At that time, her estriol and estradiol levels were normal, with low progesterone at 40 pg ml (range 100-300 pg/ml), low free testosterone at 7 pg/ml (range 8-20 pg/ml), no measurable DHEA, and relatively normal salivary cortisol samples at 8 a.m., noon, 5 p.m., and midnight. At that time, Ms. M. was being given 0.625 mg of Premarin with no progesterone.

After testing, we changed her medication to a Biest liquid suspension in a base of glycerine and a little alcohol. This was dispensed under her tongue at a dose of 0.1 ml. The concentration of the prescription was 5 mg/ml, with 20% estradiol and 80% estriol. We also prescribed 100 mg/ml natural progesterone in a base of grapeseed oil, stevia, and orange flavoring at a dose of 0.2 ml (dispensed under the tongue twice daily). We treated her DHEA deficiency with DHEA liquid suspension, 1 mg/drop at two drops twice daily. This was gradually increased to five drops twice daily.

As I recommend to all my patients, salivary testing was repeated every six to 12 months with varied dose adjustments to the sublingual suspension. In October 2002, we performed the first 24-hour urinary-hormone assay. This revealed high E1 with excessive estrogen metabolites of 16-a-hydroxyestrone and an abnormal 2-hydroxy to 16-hydrox estrone ratio. These findings placed Ms. M. at an increased risk for side effects and complications from estrogen replacement, even though the medication was "customized and natural." In this same test, DHEA, testosterone, and progesterone levels remained low.

We made appropriate dose adjustments and repeated the 24-hour urinary-hormone assay in April 2003. This test revealed low levels of all hormones due to infrequent dosing. We again modified her dose, and by November 2003 Ms. M. was feeling wonderful—with hormone levels at a safe and low level. She wrote me an enjoyable note on Nov. 22, 2003.

> "As I told you at the time of my previous refill (of HRT), you seem to have it just about right for me, and, in general I feel much as I did when I was many years younger. I think you might want to know that it has a Viagra effect. I feel fortunate that I have normal womanly feelings, but not to the extent of causing any urgency or distress".

Now how wonderful is that for 100 years young!

Fifty-three and Feeling Fine

Ms. H. is a 53-year-old female who has been a patient for just short of four years.

Initial saliva testing in May 1999 revealed no measurable progesterone, low DHEA, normal cortisol, and high estradiol, estriol and testosterone levels. Thyroid antibodies were elevated with mildly elevated TSH. Ms. H. was initially treated with 40 mg/ml of Natural Progesterone liquid suspension, 1 drop daily under her tongue; 1 mg/ml of DHEA, 1 drop in the morning; 0.05 mg of Levoxyl T4, ½ tablet daily at 10 a.m., and 15 mcg of gradual release T3 once daily at 8 a.m.

Ms. H. developed extensive inflammatory muscle and joint pain (polymalgia rheumatica) in December 1999. At that point in time, her salivary DHEA levels were still low. Instead of prescribing prednisone for polymyalgia rheumatica, we prescribed hydrocortisone (the biologically identical form of the cortisone the adrenal gland makes)—along with increased dosing of DHEA and/or 7 keto DHEA. Ms. H. remained on gradually lowered doses of hydrocortisone and DHEA through March 2002, when hydrocortisone was discontinued. She was also given pregnenalone transdermal cream (the precurosor to all adrenal hormones) 1 pump twice daily (20 mg. per pump). Her polymalgia rheumatica resolved itself without the need for further hydrocortisone. Her medication was changed to supplemental adrenal support with Isocort (glandular whole adrenal with small levels of all adrenal hormones and approximately 2 mg of naturally occurring glandular hydrocortisone per pellet). She is currently taking Isocort, 3 pellets, twice daily; no other hydrocortisone; and three sublingual sprays (5mg/spray) of DHEA each afternoon.

Female hormone replacement therapy was started in August 2003 when a 24-hour urinary hormone assay revealed no detected estrogens, low testosterone, low DHEA, and high-cortisol-related enzymes. We began replacement with a topical gel made in a base of pleuronic lecithing organogel (PLO) with 1 mg/ml of Estradiol, 4 mg/ml of Estriol, 0.5 mg/ml of Testosterone, 100 mg/ml of Progesterone with a dose of 1 ml rubbed into varied thin-skin locations daily. Due to the low DHEA levels, we measured IGF1 and revealed low IGF1 and low related growth hormone. We initiated growth-hormone-deficiency support October 2003 with pro HGH, a secretagogue that stimulates the pituitary gland to release more growth hormone and helps the pituitary to improve its release of stimulating hormones controlling adrenal, thyroid, and ovarian hormones. This was taken as two tablets diluted in water before bedtime, five days on, two days off.

As a result of this integrated hormonal support, Ms. H. had a dramatic resolution of fatigue and lifelong depression and a generalized feeling of well-being for the first time in her life, all associated with much-more-balanced female, thyroid, and adrenal hormone levels. She has stated that she is deeply grateful for the benefits balanced hormonal replacement has brought to her quality of life.

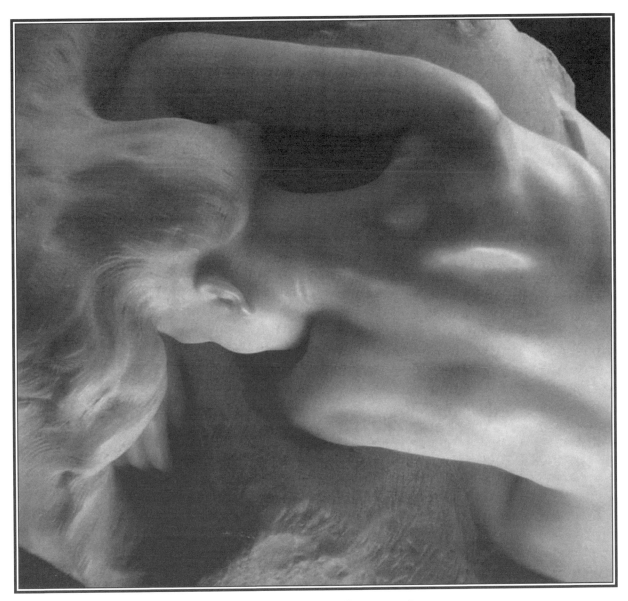

Resource Section

Resource Section

I'll conclude by reminding you that every individual's transition through menopause is unique. It is therefore very important for you to evaluate your health status individually and customize the best comprehensive approach. Some women exercise a lot, some not at all. Some will require large doses of phytonutrients to control hot flashes, and others will need unique, balanced biologically identical hormone replacement therapy. Some do great with Tricst with natural progesterone; others will need the works—thyroid support, Triest with progesterone, DHEA, testosterone, and growth-hormone secretagogues.

Your genetic individuality should absolutely be modifying the choices you and your physician are making concerning your nutritional needs, routes of delivering hormones and how safely these routes of delivery will be metabolized. Whatever approach you take, if you cross over into the arena of natural or synthetic hormone replacement therapy, you should, of course, do so with caution and with proper laboratory monitoring and physician consultation.

Hormones are potent messengers. Be sure the message your body gets is the right one, so that you can enjoy a gentle passage through menopause supporting your body, mind, and soul with a comprehensive approach of diet, exercise, stress management, mental attitude, all the essential nutrients and targeted phytonutrients, and natural hormone replacement therapy.

Following you will find a number of resources that you may find useful as you plan your approach.

Glossary

adrenal glands: Two small, triangular structures that are loosely attached to the kidneys. They have two separate parts—the outer layer, or adrenal cortex, and the adrenal medulla.

adrenaline: A neurotransmitter produced by the adrenal medulla. Known as a "fight or flight" hormone, it prepares the body for immediate action by increasing heart and metabolic rates.

amino acids: The building blocks of protein.

androgens: Male sex hormones. In women, they're produced in small amounts by the ovaries and the adrenal glands.

antioxidants: Vitamins and vitaminlike nutrients that protect the body from free-radical damage.

arteriosclerosis: Thickening of the arteries from age or high blood pressure.

asanas: Positions used in yoga.

betacarotene: The vegetable form of vitamin A.

Biest: A precompounded combination of estradiol and estriol, commonly in a 20:80 ratio.

bioidentical hormones: Hormones identical to ones naturally produced in the human body.

calcitonin: A hormone produced by the thyroid gland that lowers blood-calcium levels by causing calcium retention in bone.

carrier proteins: Substances that transport hormones through the bloodstream.

complete protein: Protein that contains all the amino acids the body needs to function properly.

conjugated horse urine: conjugated estrogens obtained from the urine of pregnant mares. The urine is extracted from mares housed on roughly 490 farms (both in Canada and the United States) and shipped to the processing plant for manufacture and marketing.

corticotropin (ACTH): A hormone that stimulates the production and release of adrenal steroids.

cortisol: The most abundant glucocorticoid produced by the adrenal cortex. It reduces inflammation, suppresses immune responses, and is secreted in greater amounts when the body is under stress.

daidzein: An isoflavone found in legumes.

dehydroepiandrosterone (DHEA): A steroid

hormone that serves as a foundation for the synthesis of other steroid hormones, including estrogen and testosterone.

diosgenin: A chemical found in wild yam that can be converted into bioidentical estrogens.

endocrine system: The bodily system composed of glands that secrete hormones directly into the blood or lymph. The major glands in the endocrine system include the pituitary, the hypothalamus, the adrenal glands, the thyroid and parathyroid, the pancreas, the ovaries, and the pineal gland.

estradiol (E2): The most potent naturally occurring estrogen in the human body.

estriol (E3): The most abundant naturally occurring estrogen in the human body.

estrogen: The umbrella term used to describe the steroid hormones produced mainly in the ovaries.

estrone (E1): Another naturally occurring estrogen in the human body. It is between E2 and E3 in potency.

follicle-stimulating hormone (FSH): A hormone produced by the pituitary gland that targets the ovaries, where it stimulates follicle growth and development. FSH also stimulates estrogen and progesterone production.

free radicals: Byproducts of the process the body uses to make energy.

genistein: A potent isoflavone found in legumes.

glucocorticoids: One of three types of steroid hormones secreted by the adrenal cortex. Glucocorticoids raise blood-sugar levels.

glycemic index: A tool that measures how foods affect blood-glucose levels.

growth factor-1 (IGF-1): An insulinlike hormone produced by the liver that promotes bone and cartilage growth, RNA formation, protein, fat, and glucose metabolism, and electrolyte balance.

growth hormone (GH): A hormone that governs normal body growth by causing liver cells to release growth factor-1.

hormones: Chemical substances produced by cells located in various glands in the body, or laboratory-created substances designed to mimic the action of naturally produced hormones.

incomplete proteins: Proteins that lack certain amino acids.

induced menopause: Immediate menopause caused by a medical or surgical intervention that removes or damages the ovaries.

isoflavones: The most potent phytoestrogens. There are more than 1,000 different types.

luteinizing hormone (LH): A hormone released by the pituitary gland that causes ovulation. It also plays a role in progesterone secretion during the second half of the menstrual cycle.

lymph: Fluid that bathes all the tissues.

macronutrients: Proteins, carbohydrates, and fats

menopause: The end of menstruation, confirmed after 12 consecutive months without a period or when the ovaries are removed or damaged.

metabolism: The ongoing, interrelated series of chemical reactions that take place in the body that provide the energy and nutrients needed to sustain life.

metabolites: Substances that are either involved in or byproducts of the metabolism of hormones.

micronutrients: Vitamins and minerals.

mineralocorticoids: One of three types of hormones produced by the adrenal cortex. They affect mineral metabolism. Aldersterone, which maintains normal blood pressure by regulating potassium, magnesium, and sodium levels in body fluids, is the most important mineralocorticoid.

natural hormone replacement therapy: Hormone therapy that uses hormones identical to those naturally produced in the body.

natural hormones: Carbon copies of the hormones naturally produced by the human body.

neurotransmitters: Brain chemicals that transmit signals that govern the action of neurons or muscle fibers.

noradrenaline: A neurotransmitter produced by the adrenal medulla. Known as a "fight or flight" hormone, it prepares the body for immediate action by increasing heart and metabolic rates.

omega-6 fatty acids: Another important type of omega fats and a good source of linoleic acid, an essential fatty acid vital to good health. It is contained in many seeds and nuts and in a number of vegetable oils.

omega-3 fatty acids: Fats that contribute to good health. They're primarily found in the oils of cold-water fish, shellfish, and sea mammals and to varying degrees in some nuts and seeds, such as flaxseed, hemp seed, soybeans, and walnuts, as well as in oils derived from them.

osteoporosis: The loss of bone mass resulting in fragile, porous bones that are prone to fractures.

peptides: One of the three chemical classes of hormones.

perimenopause: The transitional time of up to six years or more immediately prior to natural menopause (depending on when changes begin) plus one year after menopause.

phytoestrogens: Foods containing substances that have hormone-like effects.

postmenopause: All the years beyond menopause.

Premarin: A synthetic estrogen made from horse estrogen and estrone sulphate.

premature menopause: Menopause that occurs before age 40.

progestin: Synthetic progesterone.

progesterone: Often called the "feel-good hormone" due to its antidepressant and mood-enhancing effects, progesterone plays an important role in nervous system maintenance and helps balance estrogen levels. Taking progesterone with estrogen reduces estrogen dominance and reduces the chances of estrogen related endometrial cancer and other cancers caused by estrogen.

protein hormones: One of the three chemical classes of hormones.

saturated fat: A fat the molecules of which contain the maximum amount of hydrogen.

steroids: Hormones that work inside of cells to affect cell DNA and direct the production of specific enzymes and proteins.

testosterone: The primary male sex hormone, also produced in small amounts in women.

Thyroid-stimulating hormone (TSH): A hormone secreted by the pituitary gland that stimulates the synthesis and secretion of thyroid hormones.

thyroxin (T4): A hormone synthesized and secreted by the thyroid gland.

Triest: A precompounded estrogen combination that contains estrone, estradiol, and estriol in a 10:10:80 ratio.

triglycerides: The major form of fat found in the human body. They come in three forms: saturated, monounsaturated, and polyunsaturated.

triiodothyronine (T3): A hormone synthesized and secreted by the thyroid gland.

unsaturated fat: Fats that are usually liquid at room temperature, such as vegetable oils. Classed as essential fatty acids.

Appendix I

Female and Menopausal Support Products and Services

Below are additional nutritional and female-support/menopausal products and related services commonly recommended by Dr. Milner. As always, it is recommended that you first consult with a qualified professional to determine the best integrative approach to your particular situation.

Most products discussed in this book, unless otherwise noted, are available through the **Center for Natural Medicine Mail-order Dispensary** (888) 305-4288 or online at www.cnm-inc.com or www.naturalmedicineweb.com, as well as through other online and local resources.

Bezwecken Products

Isocort – Freeze-dried adrenal cortex (soluble fractionation) with DHEA and cortisol.

Phyto B – Fermented plant estrogen and progesterone with herbs.

Progon B – Fermented plant-derived progesterone and herbs.

Progonol – Fermented plant derived progesterone and herbal cream.

Osta B3 – Fermented plant estrogen and progesterone with herbs.

OstaDerm – Fermented plant-derived estrogen and progesterone cream.

Transitions – Fermented plant-derived progesterone and herbs cream.

Allvia

Transdermal hormones are available for pregnenalone, progesterone, and androstenedione in controlled pump-delivery forms.

Laboratoire Unda

Magnelevures – Each packet delivers 150 mg of highly bioavailable magnesium in the form of a fermented magnesium with,L-5-oxo-proline, glutathione, taurine, vitamins B_1, B_6, glycyrrhizin, and citric acid with natural orange flavoring. We have had excellent results using this product with people who otherwise have a hard time utilizing magnesium.

Lane Labs

3A Calcium – Highly absorbable calcium shown to remodel bone and reverse osteoporosis. This calcium supplement has been proven to rebuild bone in patients with osteoporosis just as well as the leading prescription drugs do. Three capsules contain a blend totaling 450 mg of calcium hydroxide, calcium oxide combined with an algae amino-acid extract, citric acid, gelatin, water, and glycerin.

Premier Research Lab

Coral Legend (ionized coral calcium) – This is 100%-pure coral powder with no fillers. It delivers highly ionized calcium, magnesium, and trace elements for mineral transport and absorption.

Saliva and Urine pH Testing

Martin Milner, N.D. advises his patients to regularly test and track their pH levels via single pH paper strips, which are available from local pharmacies, a number of online resources, and the Center for Natural Medicine Mail Order Dispensary; (888) 305-4288 or online at www.cnm-inc.com.

American Longevity

Dr. Milner frequently recommends the following American Longevity products:

Tangy Tangerine – Liquid vitamins, minerals, and plant-derived trace minerals, including 87 of the 90 essential nutrients, in one liquid.

Osteo Fx – Highly bioavailable liquid calcium with cofactors.

Plant-derived Minerals – Liquid plant-derived trace minerals.

EFAPlus – An essential fatty-acid blend, which contains a very good balance of omega 3, omega 6, and omega 9 fatty acids. The product contains pure uncontaminated fish oil, flax oil and borage oil, preserved with nitrogen to displace oxygen. This process dramatically retards any oxidation of the fatty acids after capsulation.

Women's Fx - A liquid menopausal support herbal formula.

Balance Fx - A formula similar to Women's FX but in capsule form.

OPCT - Green tea and grape-seed extract.

Beyond Juice – Fruit - Orange-juice powder, pineapple-juice powder, cranberry-juice powder, strawberry-juice powder, grape-juice powder, blueberry-juice powder, plum-juice powder, apricot-juice powder, cherry-juice powder, blackberry-juice powder; 900 mg. per two capsules, no calories.

Beyond Juice – Vegetable - Cabbage-juice powder, carrot-juice powder, spinach-juice powder, tomato powder, parsley-leaf powder, broccoli powder, beet-juice powder, garlic powder, brussels-sprout powder, kale powder, asparagus-juice powder, wheat-grass-juice powder, cauliflower powder; 900 mg per two capsules, no calories.

Vitale - A liquid fruit and vegetable extract it is a potent antioxidant, containing blueberry, boysenberry, alfalfa, pomegranate, green tea, bilberry, red raspberry, a blend of vegetable and fruit concentrates, broccoli, cranberry, grape-seed extract, cherry concentrate, and spinach extract, delivering an ORAC value of 1,800 per 1-oz serving.

Glyconutrients, Potent Antioxidants, and Natural-hormone Support Products Manufactured by Mannatech

Using advanced technology Mannatech extracts nutrients directly from plants and delivers them to you in convenient and effective supplements.

For further information and availability of these products go to www.cnm-inc.com.

Appendix II

Resources

American Academy of Clinical Psychology

P.O. Box 638
Niwot, CO 80544-1082
Phone: (303) 652-9154
E-mail: info@aclinp.org
Website: www.clinp.org

This organization offers referral on its website at, www.clinp.org, to qualified clinical psychologists who have passed an examination by their peers and have been certified by the American Board of Professional Psychology.

American Association for Naturopathic Physicians (AANP)

3201 New Mexico Ave., N.W. Suite 350
Washington, DC 20016
Phone: (202) 895-1392 or, toll-free (866) 538-2267
E-mail: member.services@Naturopathic.org

Website: www.naturopathic.org

This national professional society represents naturopathic physicians who are licensed (or eligible for licensing) as primary-care providers. Referrals to a naturopath in your area are available through its website at www.naturopathic.org.

The American College for Advancement in Medicine (ACAM)

23121 Verdugo Drive, Suite 204
Laguna Hills, CA 92653
Phone: (949) 583-7666 or, toll-free (800) 532-3688
E-mail: info@acam.org
Website: www.acam.org

This organization provides referrals to naturopathic physicians, who can guide you in using natural hormone therapy, on its website at www.acam.org.

The American Holistic Health Association

P.O. Box 17400
Anaheim, CA 92817-7400
Phone: (714) 779-6152
E-mail: mail@ahha
Website: www.ahha.com

This organization represents M.D.'s and D.O.'s who combine mainstream medicine with complementary therapies in their practices. It offers several resources on their website at www.ahha.com for locating qualified holistic and alternative practitioners.

American Menopause Association

350 Fifth Ave.
Suite 2822
New York, NY 10118
Phone: (212) 714-2398
Website: www.americanmenopause.org

This independent nonprofit organization provides support and assistance on all issues related to menopause. Through research, educational opportunities, and a network of volunteers, it serves as a resource for women and organizations needing information or assistance.

American Psychotherapy Association

2750 E. Sunshine
Springfield, MO 65804
Phone: (417) 823-0173
Website: www.americanpsychotherapy.com

This organization offers an online locater service through which you can choose a specialty and a state and find a listing of practitioners in your area.

American Yoga Association

P.O. Box 19986
Sarasota, FL 34276
Phone: (941) 927-4977
E-mail: info@americanyogaassociation.org
Website: www.americanyogaassociation.org

This not-for-profit organization provides high-quality instruction and educational resources for those who are interested in yoga. It is the creator of the "Easy Does it Yoga" program specially designed for seniors and the physically challenged. It offers general information about yoga and tips on choosing a yoga instructor, all of which is available on its website at www.americanyogaassociation.org.

The Association for Applied Psychophysiology and Biofeedback (AAPB)

10200 W. 44th Ave.
Suite 304
Wheat Ridge, CO 80033
E-mail: aapb@resourcenter.com
Website: www.aapb.org

Founded in 1969 as the Biofeedback Research Society this organization has as its goals to advance the understanding of biofeedback and to advance the methods used in the practice. It provides a listing of practitioners certified through the Biofeedback Certification Institute on its website America at www.aapb.org.

Center for Natural Medicine Inc.

1330 S.E. 39th Ave.
Portland, OR, 97214
Phone: (888) 305-4288
Website: www.cnm-inc.com

Most products discussed in this book are available through the Center for Natural Medicine

Mail-order Dispensary (888) 305-4288 or online at www.cnm-inc.com. Many are also available through other online and local resources.

Established in 1991 the Center is one of the oldest and largest integrated group clinics in the Pacific Northwest. This is Dr. Milner's clinic where he and other naturopathic physicians, chiropractors, acupuncturists, counselors and massage therapists practice. In addition Dr. Milner trains naturopathic physician interns, and naturopathic physician residents. CNM functions as a teaching clinic of the National College of Naturopathic Medicine.

Hypnosis Online Guide to Hypnotherapists

Website: www.hypnosisonline.com

This organization provides a collection of professional certified and registered hypnotherapists and hypnotists, organized by state and country, on its website at www.hypnosisonline.com.

International Institute of Reflexology

5650 First Ave. North
P.O. Box 12642
St. Petersburg, FL 33733-2642
Phone: (727) 343-4811
E-mail: iir@tampabay.rr.com
Website: www.reflexology-usa.net

This instructional institute teaches the Ingham Method of reflexology and provides reflexologist referrals by state on their website at www.reflexology-usa.net.

International Academy of Compounding Pharmacists

P.O. Box 1365
Sugar Land, TX 77487
Phone: (281) 933-8400 or (800) 927-4227
Fax: (281) 495-0602
Website: iacpinfo@iacprx.org

This non-profit organization offers a free referral service on its website that will locate the compounding pharmacist closest to your home zip code. Compounding pharmacists are specialists who can mix and make customized bioidentical-hormone-replacement medications in various delivery systems (pills, creams, liquids, troches, etc).

The National Acupuncture and Oriental Medicine Alliance

14637 Starr Road S.E.
Olalla, WA 98359
Phone: (253) 851-6896
E-mail: info@aomalliance.com
Website: www.acupuncturealliance.org

This organization offers online referrals to qualified practitioners matched to your geographic area on its website at www.acupuncturealliance.org.

National Certification Commission for Acupuncture and Oriental Medicine (NCCAOM)

11 Canal Center Plaza, Suite 300
Alexandria, VA 22314
Phone: (703) 548-9004
E-mail: info@nccaom.org
Website: www.nccaom.org

This not-for-profit organization has a mission of establishing, assessing, and promoting recognized standards of competence and safety in acupuncture and Oriental medicine for the protection and benefit of the public. It provides a searchable database of nationally board-certified practitioners of Oriental medicine, acupuncture, Chinese herbology, or Asian bodywork therapy on its website at www.nccaom.org.

National Guild of Hypnotists

P.O. Box 308
Merrimack, NH 03054-0308
Phone: (603) 429-9438
Website: www.ngh.net

This professional organization, established in 1951, provides online recommendations for hypnotists on its website at www.ngh.net.

North American Menopause Society (NAMS)

P.O. Box 94527
Cleveland, OH 44101
Phone: (440) 442-7550
E-mail: info@menopause.org
Website: www.menopause.org

This scientific nonprofit organization promotes women's health during mid-life and beyond through the understanding of menopause. Its website provides information on perimenopause, menopause, the health effects of estrogen loss, and other health issues affecting women.

PMU Rescue.Org

5892A S. Land Park Drive
P.O. Box 188890
Sacramento, CA 95818
Phone: (916) 429-2457
E-mail: info@uan.org
Website: www.pmurescue.org

Launched in December 2003 in reaction to the massive cuts in the Premarin industry, PMU Rescue.org is a branch of the United Animal Nations. PMU Rescue.org seeks to rescue and place mares and foals that have been left behind by the Premarin producing industry.

Reflexology Association of America

4012 Rainbow Ste,. K-PMB#585
Las Vegas, NV 89103-2059
Phone: (978) 779-0255
Website: www.reflexology-usa.org

This nonprofit organization was established to standardize and promote the professional advancement of reflexology. You can find a reflexologist by city and state, as well as internationally, on its website at www.reflexology-usa.org.

United Pegasus Foundation

120 First Ave.
Arcadia, CA 91006
Phone: (626) 279-1306
E-mail: unitedpegasus@yahoo.com
Website: www.unitedpegasus.com

The goal of this organization is to rescue pregnant mares on feed lots destined for sale to Premarin farms. In addition, UPF representatives attend horsemeat auctions to adopt foals that are a result of the Premarin farms' policies. According to 2002 statistics, there are approximately 450 Premarin farms in Canada and 50 farms in the United States, located in North Dakota, Minnesota, and Indiana, with approximately 60,000 mares.

Yoga Alliance

122 W. Lancaster Ave.
Suite 204
Reading, PA 19607-1874
Phone: (877) 964-2255 or (610) 777-0556
E-mail: info@yogaalliance.org
Website: www.yogaalliance.org

This organization established a national Yoga Teachers Registry that recognizes and promotes teachers with training that meet an established set of minimum standards.

Appendix III

Labs for Hormonal and Genomic Testing

Great Smokies Diagnostic Laboratory/Genovations™

63 Zillicoa Street
Asheville, NC 28801
Phone: (828) 253-0621 or (800) 522-4762
Fax: (828) 252-9303
Website: www.gsdl.com

This laboratory helped pioneer the field of laboratory functional testing; that is unlike traditional allopathic testing, which is concerned with the pathology of disease. Functional testing assesses the interrelationship of physiological systems in an attempt to create a more complete picture of one's health. By identifying the root causes of chronic conditions, functional testing is designed to help the practitioner develop optimal interventions to assist patients. These innovative tests cover a wide range of physiological areas, including digestive, immune, nutritional, endocrine, and metabolic functions.

Its Women's Hormonal Health Assessment includes serum/blood estrone, estradiol, estriol, 2-hydroxyestreone, 16 alpha-Hydroxyestrone, sex-hormone-binding globulin, DHEA sulphate, and testosterone. Its Comprehensive Thyroid Assessment panel includes serum/blood TSH, Free T4, Free T3, Reverse T3, anti-thyroglobulin antibodies and anti-thyroidal-peroxidase antibodies.

This laboratory also offers cutting edge genomic profile testing. By assessing genetic variations in individuals that when combined with environmental factors may increase their risk for certain disease they can assist patients and physicians in creating personalized personalized plans of preventative treatment and customized therapies for all phases of life including menopause.

Rhein Consulting Laboratories

4475 SW Scholls Ferry Road, Suite 101
Portland, OR 97225
Phone: (503) 292-1988
Fax: (503) 292-2012

Website: www.rheinlabs.com

Specializes in 24-hour-urinary-hormone panels including all estrogen metabolites. With over 28 hormones measured in the 24-hour urine specimen the type of testing this lab does is fast becoming a gold-standard in HRT monitoring surpassing saliva testing for metabolic risk factors.

Meridian Valley Laboratory

801 SW 16th, Suite 126
Renton, WA. 98055
Phone: (425) 271-8689
Fax: (425) 271-8674
Website: www.meridianvalleylab.com

Offers a 24-hour-urinary-hormone panel and salivary hormone testing.

ZRT Laboratory

1815 NW 169th Pl. Suite 5050
Beaverton, Oregon 97006
Phone: (503) 466-2445
Fax: (503) 466-1636
Website: www.zrtlab.com or www.salivatest.com

Specialize in salivary-hormone testing and employs naturopathic physicians as consultants answering health provider inquiries.

Diagnos-Techs, Inc.

Clinical and Research Laboratory
6620 S. 192nd Place, Bldg. J.
Kent, WA 98032
Phone: (800) 878-3787
Website: www.diagnostechs.com

Specialize in saliva hormone testing.

Appendix IV

Naturopathic Medical Schools of North America

Currently there are only five naturopathic medical schools in North America. A licensed naturopathic physician (N.D.) attends a four-year graduate level naturopathic medical school and is educated in all of the same basic sciences as an M.D. but also studies holistic and nontoxic approaches to therapy with a strong emphasis on disease prevention and optimizing wellness.

In addition to a standard medical curriculum, the naturopathic physician is required to complete four years of training in clinical nutrition, acupuncture, homeopathic medicine, botanical medicine, psychology, and counseling (to encourage people to make lifestyle changes in support of their personal health). A naturopathic physician takes rigorous professional board exams so that he or she may be licensed by a state or jurisdiction as a primary care general practice physician.

As of the year 2004, the following states license naturopathic physicians.

▸ Alaska

▸ Arizona

▸ California

▸ Connecticut

▸ District of Columbia

▸ Hawaii

▸ Kansas

▸ Maine

▸ Montana

▸ New Hampshire

▸ Oregon

▸ Utah

▸ Vermont

▸ Washington

▸ US Territories: Puerto Rico and Virgin Islands

▸ All Canadian Provinces

National College of Naturopathic Medicine

NCNM Main Campus
049 SW Porter Street
Portland, OR 97201
Phone: (503) 552-1555

Natural Health Center Clinic

2220 SW 1st Avenue
Portland, OR 97201
Phone: (503) 552-1551
Classical Chinese Medicine Clinic
2232 NW Pettygrove, Portland, OR 97210
Phone: (503) 552-1552
Website: www.ncnm.edu

The oldest naturopathic college in the United States where Dr. Milner has taught cardiovascular and pulmonary medicine since 1986. NCNM also offers a masters degree program in Oriental Medicine.

Bastyr University

14500 Juanita Dr. NE
Kenmore, WA 98028-4966
Phone: (425) 823-1300
Fax: (425) 823-6222 fax
Website: www.bastyr.edu

The largest alternative medicine academic institution in the United States offering other programs in addition to naturopathic medical education.

Southwest College of Naturopathic Medicine

2140 E. Broadway Rd.
Tempe, AZ 85282
Phone: (480) 858-9100
Website: www.scnm.edu

University of Bridgeport College of Naturopathic Medicine

Health Science Center
60 Lafayette Street
Bridgeport, CT 06604
Phone: (800) EXCEL UB ext. 4108
E-mail: natmed@bridgeport.edu
Website: www.bridgeport.edu/pages/3240.asp

The Canadian College of Naturopathic Medicine

1255 Sheppard Ave. E.,
Toronto, ON M2K 1E2 Canada
Phone: (866) 241-2266 (toll free)
Website: www.ccnm.edu

Bibliography

Much of the information in this book was obtained through medical journals, books, medical articles in popular publications, Internet sources, and research abstracts obtained through computer searches of medical databases. Below is a partial listing of those resources.

Adelson, Harry N.D. "The Naturopathic Approach to the Treatment of Menopause," Menopause Online: www.menopause-online.com

Amato, P., S. Christophe, and P.L. Mellon. "Estrogenic activity of Herbs Commonly Used as Remedies for Menopausal Symptoms,". Menopause 200s Mar-Apr: 9(2):145-50.

Anderson J.and S.Garner. "Effects of Soy Isoflavones on Bone,". Nutr Aspects Osteoporosis 1998; 172-179 (Proc. Symp. 1997)

Anti-aging and Cardiovascular Health Center Inc. Information online at www.anti-agingandcv.com

Armstrong, David. "Data Increases Doubts About Hormone Therapy," Wall Street Journal, March 13, 2003.

Balk, Judith. "Mind-body Approaches to Menopausal Symptoms," Alternative Medicine Alert, Feb. 2003.

Bauer, Joy. The Complete Idiot's Guide to Total Nutrition, Third Edition. New York: Alpha Books, 2003

Begley, Sharon. "A Bit Under the Gun During the Holidays? Well, It's Good for You," Wall Street Journal, Dec. 26, 2003.

Boyles, Salynn. "Low Estrogen Linked to Heart Disease, Sex Hormone May Protect Women Prior to Menopause," WebMD Medical News, Feb. 4, 2003

"Consensus Opinion of The North American Menopause Society, The Role of Isoflavones in Menopausal Health:," Menopause: The Journal of The North American Menopause Society, Vol. 7, No. 4, pp.215-229.

"Consensus Opinion of the North American Menopause Society: The role of Calcium in Peri- and Postmenopausal

Women," <u>Menopause: The Journal of the North American Menopause Society</u>, Vol. 8, No. 2, pp. 84-95.

Davis, Jeanie. "Breast Cancer Risk Subsides After HRT." WebMD Medical News, Dec. 2, 2002

"Soy's Menopause Benefits Questioned, Seems to Help Hot Flashes, but May Be Placebo Effect," WebMD Medical News, Oct. 4, 2002

Dean, Carolyn. <u>Menopause Naturally</u>. Los Angeles: Keats Publishing, 1999

DeNoon, Daniel. "Most Women Not Quitting HRT, but Many Who Stop Estrogen Don't Get Other Bone Protection," WebMD Medical News, Jan. 13, 2003

Edelberg, David. "Supplement Recommendations for Menopause," Online at www.wholehealthmd.com

The Endocrine Society. "Androgens in women." Online at www.androgensinwomen.com

FDA Statement on the Results of the Women's Health Initiative. www.fda.gov.

Ferlow Brothers. Product information on wild yam. Online at www.ferlowbrothers.com/wildyam_meno.htm

Francina, Suza. <u>Yoga and the Wisdom of Menopause: A Guide to Physical, Emotional, and Spiritual Health at Midlife and Beyond</u>. Deerfield Beach, Fl.: Health Communications Inc., 2003.

Gaffney B.T., H.M. Hugel, and P.A. Rich, "Panax Ginseng and Eleutherococcus Senticosus May Exaggerate an Already Biphasic Repsonse to Stress via Inhibition of Enzymes Which Limit the Binding of Stress Hormones to Their Receptors," Med Hypotheses 2001; 56(5):567-572

Gale Encyclopedia of Alternative Medicine

Gardner, Amanda. "Natural Hormone Leads to Less Bleeding," www.drkoop.com, Nov. 1, 2002

Gittleman, Ann Louise. <u>Before The Change: Taking Care of Your Perimenopause</u>. San Francisco: Harper Collins, 1998

Glazier, M., Gina Bowman, and A. Marjorie, "A Review of the Evidence for the Use of Phytoestrogens as a Replacement for Traditional Estrogen Replacement Therapy," <u>Arch Intern Med</u>. 2001;161

Gobbi M., F. Dalla Valle, C. Ciapparelli, et. al., "Hypericum Perforatum L. Extract Does Not Inhibit 5-HT Transporter in Rat-brain Cortex," Arch Pharmacol 1999; 360:262-269

Goodman, MT, McDuffied K, Kolonel LN, Terada K, Donlon TA, Wilkens LR, Guo C, Le Marchand L, "Case-control Study of Ovarian Cancer and Polymorphisms in Genes Involved in Catecholestrogen Formation and Metabolism," Cancer Epidemiol Biomarkers Prev, 2001;10:209-216

Gordon, Serena. "Alternative Medicine a Mixed Bag for Menopause," HealthScoutNews. Online at ABCnews.go.com/sections/living/Healthology/HS_AlternativeMenopause021119.html

Greenberg, Beth. "If It's Not PMS, It Might Be Perimenopause," Boston Globe, April 15, 2003.

Harrar, Sari. "Stop Your Hormone Replacement Therapy? Read This First!" Online at www.prevention.com/cda/feature2002/0,4780,3865,00.html

"Menopause: Herbs That Can Ease The Transition" (excerpted from Herbs for Health magazine), Health World Online, www.healthy.net

"Remedies for Menopause," Online at www.holistic-online.com

Hoegler, Nancy. "Research Reviews: St. John's Wort Relieves Menopause Symptoms," Herb World News Online, www.herbs.org

Hübner W.D, S. Lande, H. Podzuweit. "Hypericum Treatment of Mild Depressions with Somatic Symptoms," Journal of Geriatric Psychiatry and Neurology 1994;7 (suppl. 1): S12-S14

Hudson, Tori, N.D. "Osteoporosis: Natural Therapies in Prevention and Treatment." "Women's Encyclopedia of Natural Medicine"

"Hormone Replacement Therapy: Benefits, Risks, and Options," Integrative Medicine, 2003;2 (1)

Huntley, Alyson, E. Ernst. "A Systematic Review of the Safety of Black Cohosh," Menopause: The Journal of the North American Menopause Society. Vol. 10, No. 1, pp. 58-64.

Kalyn, Wayne, ed. The Healing Power of Vitamins, Minerals and Herbs. Readers Digest, 1999

Kamen, Betty. Hormone Replacement Therapy, Yes or No? How to Make an Informed Decision About Estrogen,

Progesterone and Other Strategies for Dealing With PMS, Menopause and Osteoporosis. Novato, CA: Nutrition Encounter, 1996

Kirchheimer, Sid, "Depression, Early Perimenopause Linked, Risk Highest in Those Currently Taking Medication," WebMD Medical News, Jan. 13, 2003

Kling, Jim. Once Promising Future of HRT Dwindles. WebMD Medical News, October 23, 2002.

Kolata, Gina. "No Gain Outweighing Risk Found in Hormone Therapy." New York Times, March 17, 2003.

"Race to Fill Void in Menopause-drug Market," The New York Times, Sept. 1, 2002

"Replacing Replacement Therapy," The New York Times, Oct. 27, 2002.

"Why Hormone Studies Led to Different Findings is Still a Mystery," The New York Times, April 28, 2003.

Komesaroff, P.A., C.V. Black, V. Cable, and K. Sudhir, "Effects of Wild Yam Extract on Menopausal Symptoms, Lipids and Sex Hormones in Healthy Menopausal Women," Climacteric 2001;4(2):144-150

Krapp, Kristine M. and, Jacqueline Longe,

eds. The Gale Encyclopedia of Alternative Medicine. Detroit: Gale Group, 2000

Lark, Susan M. The Menopause Self Help Book: A Woman's Guide to Feeling Wonderful for the Second Half of Her Life. Berkeley, CA: Celestial Arts, 1990

Liu J., et al., "Evaluation of Estrogenic Activity of Plant Extracts for the Potential Treatment of Menopausal Symptoms." J Agric Food Chem 2001 May: 49(5):2472-2479

Love, Susan M. Dr. Susan Love's Menopause & Hormone Book. New York: Three Rivers Press, 2003

Mann, Denise, "NAMS: New Recommendations Reaffirm That Symptom Relief Is Prime Indication for Hormone Replacement Therapy," DG News, Oct. 4, 2002

Matsui A, Ikeda T, Enomoto K, Hosoda K, Nakashima H, Omae K, Watanabe M, Hibi T, Kitajima M, "Increased Formation of Oxidative DNA Damage, 8-hydroxyl-2'-deoxyguanosine in Human Breast Cancer Tissue and Its Relationship to GSTP1 and COMT Genotypes," Cancer Lett 2000;151:87-95

McCaleb, Rob, "Research Reviews: St. John's Wort Equivalent to World's Best-selling

Antidepressant," Herb World News Online, www.herbs.org

Miller, K.A., "Androgen Deficiency in Women," J Clin Endocrinol Metab 2001;86:2395-2401

Menopause Core Curriculum Study Guide, 2nd Edition. 2002, North American Menopause Society

Menopause Online. Information on HRT, perimenopause, herbal remedies, and more. Online at www.menopause-online.com

Morien, Krista, "Research Reviews: Safety of St. John's Wort versus Antidepressant Drugs," Herb World News Online, www.herbs.org

MSNBC staff and wire reports, "Estrogen Hikes Ovarian-cancer Risk," MSNBC, July 16, 2002

Murray, GI, Melvin WT, Greenlee WF, Burke MD, Regulation, Function and Tissue Specific Expression of Cytochrome P450 CYP1B1," Ann. Rev. Pharmacol Taxicol 2001;41:297-316

National Center for Health Statistics, Division of Data Services. Online: www.cdc.gov/nchs/releases/03news/lifeex.htm

Neel, Joe. The Marketing of Menopause. National Public Radio, Aug. 8, 2002

Nestel P.J., et al.,Pomeroy S, Kay S, "Isoflavones From Red Clover Improve Systemic Arterial Compliance but Not Plasma Lipids in Menopausal Women," Journal of Clinical Endocrinology and Metabolism 1999; 84(3): 895-898

North American Menopause Society. Online: www.menopause.org.

O'Shea, Tim, "Hormone Replacement Therapy: When Is It Necessary (Part 1)," Online: www.mercola.com.

Osumex. Product information, information on lignans. Online: www.osumex.com

People for the Ethical Treatment of Animals. Information on hormone replacement therapy, naturopathic approach, traditional and alternative treatments. Online:www.menopauseonline.com

"Role of Progestogen in Hormone Therapy for Postmenopausal Women: Position Statement of The North American Menopause Society," Menopause: The Journal of The North American Menopause Society. Vol. 10, No. 2, pp. 113-132.

Randolph, John F. Jr. and Lorraine Dennerstein, "Female Androgen Deficiency Syndrome: A Hard Look at a Sexy Issue," Contemporary Issues in Ob/Gyn & Women's Health. Online: www.medscape.com

Reuters Health Information, Jan. 13, 2003, "Depression Linked to Early Onset of Perimenopause," reporting on findings published in the Jan. 13, 2003 issue of the Archives of General Psychiatry

Reginster J.Y., A. Kvasz, O. Bruyere, Y. Henrotin. "Is There Any Rationale for Prescribing Hormone Replacement Therapy (HRT) to Prevent or to Treat Osteoarthritis?," Osteoarthritis Cartilage 2003 Feb;11(2):87-91.

Rosenberg S., Jenkins D.J., Diamandis E.P., "Effects of Natural Products and Nutraceuticals on Steroid Hormone-related Gene Expression," Clin Chim Acta 2001 Oct;312(1-2):213-219

Rostler, Suzanne, "HRT, Drinking Milk Tied to Cancer Hormone in Women," Reuter's News Service, Sept. 10, 2002

Sanderoff, Brian T. "Hormone Replacement Therapy – an Idea Whose Time Has Passed. Your Prescription for Health," Online Holistic Pharmacy, Online: www.prescription4health.com

Seidl M.M., D.E. Stewart, "Alternative Treatments for Menopausal Symptoms, Systematic Review of Scientific and Lay Literature," Canadian Family Physician; 1998, 44: 1299-1308

Sheehy, Gail. The Silent Passage. New York: Pocket Books, a division of Simon & Schuster Inc., 1991

2002 Sleep in America Poll. Washington DC: National Sleep Foundation; 1998. Accessible at www.sleepfoundation.org/2002poll.html

Spake, Amanda, "The Menopausal Marketplace." Online: www.usnews.com

Sparrowe, Linda. The Women's Book of Yoga & Health: A Lifelong Guide to Wellness. Boston: Shambala Publications Inc., 2002

A Study of Women's Health Across the Nation (SWAN), information on early menopause. Online at www.remifemin.com/article_022.asp.

Tanner, Lindsey. "Health & Science: Doubt over Hormone Supplements Debated as Menopause Specialists Meet," AP Online, Oct. 3, 2002

Taylor, Maida, "Phyto-Estrogens," HCRC FAQ Sheet. Online: www.hcrc.org.

Tesch, Bonnie, "New Studies Question the Use of Herbs for Menopause Relief," Online: http://healthlink.mcw.edu

"Black Cohosh May Reduce Menopausal Symptoms," Online: http://healthlink.mcw.edu.

Tilgner, Sharol, N.D., "Phytoestrogens,". Online: www.planetherbs.com

U.S. Preventive Services Task Force., "Postmenopausal Hormone Replacement Therapy for Primary Prevention of Chronic Conditions: Recommendations and Rationale," Annals of Internal Medicine, 19 November 2002, Volume 137, Number 10.

Vliet, Elizabeth Lee. Screaming to Be Heard: Hormonal Connections Women Suspect and Doctors Still Ignore. M. Evans & Co., 2001

Wallach, Joel and Ma Lan, Dead Doctors Don't Lie. Legacy Communication Group, Franklin, TN: 1999,

Wallach, Joel and Ma Lan, Let's Play Doctor. Wellness Publication LLC, 1989-2000

Wallach, Joel and Ma Lan, Let's Play Herbal Doctor. Wellness Publications, LLC 2001

Wallach, Joel and Ma Lan, Rare Earth, Forbidden Cures. Double Happiness Publishing Co., 1994-1996

Walters David D., et al., "Effects of Hormone Replacement Therapy and Antioxidant Vitamin Supplements on Coronary Atherosclerosis in Postmenopausal Women, A Randomized Controlled Trial," JAMA 2002;288:2,432-2,440.

Warren, Barbour. Phytoestrogens and the Risk of Breast Cancer. Program on breast cancer and environmental risk factors, Cornell University

Williamson, J. A. White, A. Hart, E. Ernst, "Randomized Controlled Trial of Reflexology for Menopausal Symptoms." BJOG. 2002 Sep; 109 (9):1050-1,055

Winslow, Ron and Geeta Anand, "Latest Hormone-Drug Study Adds Both Clarity, Confusion to Issue," Wall Street Journal, July 23, 2002

Wright, Jonathan V., and John Morgenthaler, "Natural Hormone Replacement For Women Over 45," Petaluma, CA.: Smart Publications, 1997

Zava, D.T., C.M. Dollbaum, M. Blen, "Estrogen and Progestin Bioactivity of Foods, Herbs, and Spices,". Proc Soc Exp Biol Med 1998 Mar;217(3):369-378

Index

and stress, 152
and sugar in diet, 117
and Vitamin E, 139
Diabetic neuropathy, and evening-primrose oil, 176
Diagnos-Techs, Inc., 214
Diarrhea, and herbal remedies, 175
Diet
and age-related hormonal changes, 34
and free radicals, 134
and osteoporosis, 10
poor, and gene expression, 90-91
recommendations for, **120-121**
Dietary supplement, legal definition of, 169
Dihydrotestosterone (DHT), 22
and SSRIs, 42
Dioscorides, 181
Diosgenin, 201
in wild yam, 67-68, 182
Dipstick, urine, and high-protein diet, 102
Discharge, heavy vaginal, homeopathic remedies for, 184
Discomfort during sex, as symptom, 46-47
Discorea villosa. *See* Wild yam
Disease, and gene expression, 90-91
Dizziness, as side-effect of herbal remedies, 181
DNA (deoxyribonucleic acid)
nuclear, and testosterone, 23
structure of, *86*, *87*
DOE. *See* Department of Energy
Dong quai (Angelica sinensis), as natural remedy, **174-175**
Dopamine, 89
and physical exercise, 146
Drinking, and osteoporosis, 10
Drinks
cool, as treatment for hot flashes, 44
hot, as trigger for hot flashes, 45
DRIs (dietary reference intakes), 125
Drugs, and gene expression, 90-91
DRV (daily reference value). *See* RDA
Dry eyes, as symptom, 40
Dry mouth, as side-effect of herbal remedies, 181
Dryness, vaginal. *See* Vaginal dryness
Dry skin

and declining testosterone, 47
as symptom, 40, 41
Vitamin E for, 138
DV (daily value). *See* RDA

E
EAR (estimated average requirement), for micronutrients, 126
Economic status. *See* Socioeconomic status
Eczema, and evening-primrose oil, 176
EFAs. *See* Fatty acids, essential
Eggs (human)
implantation of, 7
in menstrual cycle, 6-7
Eggs (poultry), and omega-3 fatty acids, 107
Electrolyte balance, and growth-factor-1, 19
ELSI (ethical, legal, and social issues), of the Human Genome Project, 87
Emotional issues, 11
exercise and, 144
and nutrition, 95-96
Endocrine system, 201
components of, 16
feedback loops in, 17
and pituitary gland, 6
Endometrial cancer. *See* Cancer, endometrial
Endometrial hyperplasia, 29
Endometriosis, and hormonal problems, 9
Endorphins
and acupuncture/acupressure, 156
and physical exercise, 144, 146
Energy level, declining, and declining testosterone, 47
English valerian. *See* Valerian
Enterodiol, 104
Enterolactone, 104
Environment (personal), and stress, 152-153
Enzymes, natural, in honey, 114
EP. *See* Epinephrine
Epilepsy
and early onset, 8
and evening-primrose oil, 176
Epinephrine (EP), *25*, **25-26**, 89
vs. norepinephrine (NE), 26
and stress, 152

Equal, as sugar substitute, 115
Equilin
in conjugated estrogen drugs, 67-68
patentable, 66
Esclim, *61*
Estrace (tablets and cream), *28*, *61*
Estraderm, *28*, *61*
Estradiol (E2), *23*, *27*, *28*, 201
as bioidentical (natural) hormone, 67
dehydroepiandrosterone (DHEA) and, 22
diagnostic testing for, 49
in food, FDA approval of, 100
natural, 71-72
in natural hormone therapy, 71-72
prescription transdermal, *61*
and testosterone, 23, *23*
Estratab, *61*
Estratest, *28*
Estring, *61*
Estriol (E3), *27*, *28*, *71*, 201
as bioidentical (natural) hormone, 67
diagnostic testing for, 49
in natural hormone therapy, 71-72
Estrogen dominance, 28
Estrogen receptors
in arterial walls, and hot flashes, 44
and phytoestrogens, 103, 167, 175
Estrogen replacement
and folic-acid levels, 138
and wild yam, 183
Estrogens, 17, *27*, **27-30**, *28*, 201
conjugated equine (Premarin), *61*
converted from testosterone, 22-23
in cycling hormone therapy, 81
declining, and sexual dysfunction, 46-47
and hot flashes, 44
in menstrual cycle, 6-7, 49
natural, *vs.* phytoestrogens, 103
in natural hormone therapy, 71-72
as neurotransmitter regulator, 42
oral
list of, *61*
and SHBG, 47
physical exercise and, 145
role of, in body, 29

About the Author

Key Credentials

Martin Milner, N.D.

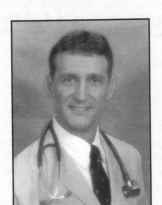

▶ CEO and Medical Director, Center for Natural Medicine Inc., Portland, OR.

▶ Professor, Cardiovascular and Pulmonary Medicine, National College of Naturopathic Medicine, Portland, OR.

▶ Medical Advisor, Health Sciences Institute, Baltimore, MD

Dr. Milner received his N.D. in 1983 from National College of Naturopathic Medicine (NCNM) Portland Oregon. He has remained at his alma mater for the past eighteen years as Professor of Cardiovascular and Pulmonary Medicine. Dr. Milner is also the CEO and medical director of the Center for Natural Medicine (CNM), Inc. Established in 1991, CNM is the first and one of the largest ongoing, integrated healthcare facilities in the Northwest.

The Heart and Lung Wellness program is the newest addition in Dr. Milner's professional life, linking his identities as professor and doctor. This exciting new program provides a clinical training ground for 16-24 fourth year medical students and resident doctors, supervised by Dr. Milner. This experience engages medical students and patients in collaborative, complimentary and alternative health care of cardiovascular, pulmonary disease and primary care conditions. In this capacity CNM functions as a teaching clinic of NCNM.

Dr. Milner is well published with texts, medical journal articles and studies in endocrinology, cardiology, pulmonology, oncology, and environmental medicine. In July 2005 an article will be published in the *International Journal of Pharmaceutical Compounding* guiding physicians and compounding pharmacists in the management of hypothyroidism using his protocol of gradual released compounded thyroid replacement. His feature article in *Alternative and Complementary Therapies* (June 2002) entitled "Natto and Its Active Ingredient Nattokinase." introduced the use of Nattokinase into the United States. Dr. Milner served as the primary consulting physician for Judith Sach's book <u>Natural Medicine for Heart Disease</u>. Also to his credit are "Wilson's Syndrome and T3 therapy – A Clinical Guide to Safe and Effective Patient Management" in the *International Journal of Pharmaceutical Compounding* Vol. 3 No. 5, Sept/Oct 1999, p. 344-349 and the co-authoring of

chapter 14 in <u>An Alternative Medicine Definitive Guide to Cancer</u> by J. Diamond and W.L. Cowden.

Dr. Milner has been the medical advisor for the Health Sciences Institute (H.S.I.) and its publications since 1996. H.S.I.'s monthly newsletter circulates to approximately 100,000 subscribers around the world introducing cutting edge, breakthrough and well research nutraceuticals to the readership. He has delivered a compelling presentation titled "ADDSOIL- 7 Keys to Optimal Health" available as a self help resource guide with companion audio tapes through Health Sciences Institute, Agora Publications, 1999.

Dr. Milner is a dynamic speaker with a bachelors and masters degree in education from the University of Rhode Island. He brings a fresh and enjoyable approach to his lectures using the latest in computerized technology. He has lectured extensively for over 20 years nationally and internationally, to physicians groups and public audiences alike.